To CRSF

(castle ~mom

MW01259245

ADVANCE PRAISE

Unforgivable is a compelling story about the challenges that people face and the difficulties they endure. It is a tribute to the will to live and fight against almost insurmountable odds. This very human story is one of love and hate, positive and negative emotions.

—Rabbi Bruce Aft, Adjunct professor, George Mason University, Fairfax, VA

"War is hell." So goes the saying about geo-political warfare. But so is one's private war. This story tells the story of two brave young boys growing up in Nazi-occupied Holland, each warring against internal and external enemies, only to see much later that, somehow, they survived and overcame the extremes of abuse, abandonment, and apathy of those that should have provided them everyday protection and care. Frits and Jan will find their way into your heart, and you will not only be wiser about the unsung casualties of warfare but also better for it.

—David Case, Christian Studies teacher, Trinity Christian School, Fairfax, VA

Through the horror of war and unspeakable abuse as a child, Frits' story is poignant, engaging, and compellingly told by his beloved daughter. His long and painful journey led to forgiveness and, finally, to saying "yes" to the One who forgives the unforgivable.

—The Right Reverend John Guernsey (ret), Anglican Church in North America, VA

WOW for this book!! I was utterly immersed in Frits's story. So moving! So infuriating! So haunting! So inspiring! *Unforgivable* is truly a timely book. We are now hearing about the horrors the Native Americans suffered in both American and Canadian boarding schools. Unfortunately, this is nothing new. I strongly recommend *Unforgivable*.

—Bruce Hann, Emeritus Professor of Literature and Rhetoric, DMACC, Ankeny, IA

In this emotional and heartfelt story, author Caroline Crocker brings the reader into the traumatic life of her father. Based on letters and other documents sharing his actual experiences, the author provides details of the day-to-day journey that shaped her father into the man he became. I read and cried, read and cried. I was amazed at how he found joy in simple things. A great read.

—Melissa Henderson, Award award-winning author, Charleston, SC

In today's tumultuous times, many feel the world has never seen darker days. But those who lived through the horrors of the Second World War surely felt the same as they watched the world crumble around them. As a serious scholar who has done extensive historical research, Caroline Crocker's book provides a poignant reminder that humanity has persevered through unimaginable adversity. Frits's inspirational journey shows the world not only what we have overcome but what we can overcome.

—The Reverend Canon David Roseberry, Executive Director, LeaderWorks, Canon for Mission, the Anglican Church in North America, Plano, TX

Caroline Crocker's engaging telling of the story of her father's traumatic life invites the reader not only to reflect on the many challenges he faced but also to consider the nature of forgiveness, which it raises. It's a great way to think about such weighty matters, and I recommend it warmly.

—Reverend Dr. Justyn Terry, Vice Principal and Academic Dean, Wycliffe Hall, Oxford, England

I highly recommend this book as it truly draws you to the horror of life at that time while demonstrating that God's love is still greater than the depravity of humanity.

—The Reverend Dr. Johannes W H van der Bijl, SAMS-USA Missionary, Chaplain, Langham Author, Heiloo, The Netherlands

This is a wonderful book. The dialogue is filled with compassion and wit. Often, I could not read any more in a sitting because I had to take a break from the hardships of Frits and his brother. It is incredible that they were able to have anything like normal lives after their treatment. I intend to reread the book.

—Dr. Mary Vander Maten, Dean of Math, Science and Engineering (ret.), Northern Virginia Community College, Annandale, VA

Such a personal and profound story! I feel privileged to have read it and am struck by the character and endurance of Frits. What a man! This book is a treasure.

—Susan Alexander Yates, Author and Speaker, Falls Church, VA

UNFORGIVABLE

_____

THROUGH A CHILD'S EYES

I. CAROLINE CROCKER

ISBN 978-1-957970-10-3 (ebook)
ISBN 978-1-957970-12-7 (paperback)
ISBN 978-1-957970-11-0 (hardcover)
Publisher: RamblingRuminations, Fairfax, VA, USA

Unforgivable is a sidequel to *Brave Face: The Inspiring WWII Memoir of a Dutch/German Child,* which tells the story of Meta's childhood.

Copyright © I. Caroline Crocker, January 10, 2024

Cover image: GRAPHIXMUNNA

The stories in this book were inspired by actual events in the life of Frits Evenbly. Most of the names belong to real people, the majority of whom are deceased. Every effort has been made to portray these people faithfully. The dialogue and some names are products of the author's imagination.

Illustrations are primarily from the author's family album but also include some public-domain photographs.

Book website: https://unforgivable.website

Author blog: https://ramblingruminations.com

YouTube playlist: https://tinyurl.com/fritsevenblij

All Rights Reserved. No part of this publication may be reproduced or transmitted in any form or by any means, electronic or mechanical, including photocopy, recording, or any other information storage and retrieval system, without prior written permission from the publisher.

CONTENTS

READER INFORMATION

This book is about the lives of people who are no longer with us. I have drawn some of the content from what they told my mother and me. Their letters, diaries, papers, and memoirs provided additional insights. Next, I conducted historical research and read articles published online. The remainder is imaginative speculation. Having said that, throughout the book, I've been careful only to include those incidents that actually happened. Thus, this is a true story—mostly.

Please be aware that, in the interest of geographical authenticity, I included words and phrases in different languages. There is a glossary of foreign language words to assist readers who don't speak or read French, German, and Dutch. There's also an appendix to help readers keep track of the various characters.

For the sake of historical authenticity, I included words that may offend. Of course, it's wrong to refer to servants as "garçon," but it's what those living in the Belgian Congo in the 1930s did. Similarly, Dutch people living under occupation did refer to their occupiers as "*Moffen*." I don't commend these practices, but I put the words in this book anyway. Other Dutch swear words are also sprinkled throughout the book because that's how my father spoke. He lives through these pages.

Dedicated to my beloved father, Frits Evenbly,
and his brother, Jan.

Also, to Frederik Evenblij, the grandfather I never met,
and Keetie van Zanten, Dad's good friend.

Dad, your life helped me to understand my heavenly Father's
love. You gave me my passion for teasing out problems and learning
how things work. You gave me the confidence to keep going simply
because someone in this world understood and believed in me.
I love you, Dad. I always will.

Oom Jan, I wish I could have known you better,
but am very grateful for the few times we could meet.

Opa, I never knew you, but the love in your letters to Dad
warms my heart.

Keetie, Dad never forgot you;
because of him, you have a place in my heart.
Although none of your family survived the Holocaust,
I hope this book will ensure that you will be remembered.

All of your outstanding contributions made it possible to write
this book about your lives, and I am grateful.

To forgive is

to set a prisoner free

and to discover

the prisoner was you.

--Corrie ten Boom

FOREWORD

When I met Frits Evenbly in his last years, I could tell he was quite the character—especially by the effect of his personality and giftings on his daughter (and my friend) Caroline. I loved seeing how he loved and supported Caroline in *her* personality and giftings.

What I didn't know was *why* he was quite the character. Until I read *Unforgivable.*

His childhood traumas, one stacked on another in ways that made me wince, had scooped him out until he was bigger on the inside than he was on the outside. I literally did wince as I read portions of his story; my heart wrenched with compassion and horror for what he experienced as a boy.

I had heard about abuses in war-torn communities, but *Unforgivable* educated me in ways I will never forget without being gratuitous. Just . . . heart-moving.

As I read it, I wanted to know how the story ended, but I didn't want it to end. I love books like that.

Now, I know that meeting Frits wasn't just a pleasant encounter for me but a great honor. I'm confident you will wish that you, too, had the opportunity to meet the man.

Sue Bohlin
Writer and Speaker for Probe Ministries

PREFACE

Soon after the publication of *Brave Face: The Inspiring WWII Memoir of a Dutch/German Child*, my mother, Meta, and I heard an outcry. "We want more!"

I wanted to provide that by writing about my father, Frits's, life, but it seemed unlikely I could. After all, it would be virtually impossible to gather the necessary information. He passed in October 2017. But then, Meta unearthed the letters his father wrote to him, as well as the documents my parents saved from their early life. I reread the brief account of Frits's childhood that he wrote for their 50th anniversary and what he wrote for the 60th. My cousin sent me a document her father, Frits' brother, Jan, penned about his life. An online acquaintance provided me with research on the children's home where Frits and Jan spent much of their childhood. I bought and translated the out-of-print book that Frits's mother, Rita, wrote about her wartime experiences. Gradually, this book took shape.

It has been a fascinating journey. I've spent many hours immersed in historical research, trying to tease out what really happened in that little town of Driebergen. So many tantalizing clues, but elucidating all the facts, something I find very important, has proven impossible. Therefore, I've written what I'm reasonably sure happened and left the rest for you to think about.

I've enjoyed trying to get into the heads of the various characters in this book. Why did Rita do what seems totally repugnant? Why did Frits and Jan react to their life circumstances like they did? How must Frits's Jewish cousin have felt, seeing all that was happening around her? What were the overly strict nurses in the children's home even thinking? I found my research into the possible thought processes of the various characters totally engrossing.

It has been a testing journey. Much of Frits's story is deeply disturbing and, frankly, depressing. To make a book come to life, the writer must live it. And so, I did. Conventional wisdom is that authors should write every day. I couldn't do that simply because spiraling down into depression does not help one write! Frits had to live his story every day without a break; I did not. And I am grateful.

It has been a very worthwhile journey. You see, despite his shockingly tough childhood, Frits successfully provided for and raised five children. His and Meta's marriage was challenging at times, but they celebrated their 60th wedding anniversary only half a year before he died. He passed on so many good things to me, not the least of which is the confident knowledge that he loved and believed in me. I was amazing in his eyes.

Frankly, Frits's successful life made me curious. How did he do it? Why didn't he spend his life on antidepressants and in therapy (not that those are bad things)? A conversation with Meta provided what I suspect was at least a partial answer. I believe anyone who has ever been mistreated or experienced trauma can find a vital message in Frits's story. Yup. That's everyone. This book is for everybody. But you'll have to read it to find out what that message is.

I. Caroline Evenbly Crocker, PhD
caroline@ramblingruminations.com

1

THE MURDERS

"Frits, stop your ridiculous tinkering!" Zuster (Sister) Dermout's harsh voice made me jump. "We're nearly out of firewood. Go now. Find some before it gets dark."

I looked outside. The sun was low in the sky, but I knew better than to argue. At least later, the moon might light my way. That is if the clouds would cooperate.

"Come on, Jan." I shoved my beloved screwdriver into my pocket before grasping my younger brother's hand with all the authority an eight-year-old can muster. "I'll need your help." I lined our shoes with newspaper so our toes wouldn't freeze, then struggled into my too-small, threadbare coat. I put my hat over Jan's rioting blond curls and pulled his coat sleeves down to cover his hands.

My spirits lifted when we reached *het bos* (the forest). There was something magical about the trees pushing their long fingers into the sky, the fragrances that changed with the season, and the total isolation from the hustle and bustle of Driebergen, the little town in the center of the Netherlands where we lived.

"Wait for me!" Jan pled as, breathless, he struggled through the snow.

"Here, help me pull." I placed my little brother's hand on the wagon's handle, knowing full well that now I'd be pulling him as well as it. Because the villagers would have harvested everything from the edges of the woods, we had to walk further, and time was short if we were to finish before dark.

"This should be far enough," I muttered. "Do what I'm doing, Jan." Using my foot, I pushed aside the snow before picking up sticks and branches.

"I'm cold!' Jan's teeth were chattering.

1

"Well, work faster! That'll help."

Once we'd found all we could in one place, we moved to the next until we were a long way from *het kindertehuis* (the children's home). That's where we lived with over 30 children, all of whom were cared for by two nurses, known to us as "sisters."

"Okay, that should be enough. Let's go." Suddenly, I froze, arrested by bangs echoing through the trees.

"Frits, what's that?" My six-year-old brother's voice trembled as his blue eyes scanned our surroundings.

"Guns! Run!" The sisters had warned us about this. I knew that when we hear gunfire, we should go to the nearest house. So, pulling our fully laden wagon with one hand and my brother with the other, I ran out of the woods and into a tree-lined lane.

The houses along this street had tiny front gardens, each bordered by a rose hedge.
I opened my mouth to tell Jan we should go into the first house, where the door already stood open. Guttural shouting changed my mind. Germans! We halted abruptly.

Jan knew to keep quiet, but just in case, I pulled his trembling body close to mine and put my icy hand over his mouth. Both of us crouched behind the hedge.

There in the front yard were three Nazi soldiers in woolen uniforms and shiny black boots, their machine guns slung over their shoulders. A stone-faced German with narrowed eyes came out of the home, dragging a ragged Dutch man forward by his arm.

"No, no, we were just having dinner together!" The wild-eyed man glanced over his shoulder. "Go back in, Hylke. Hide!"

The soldier responded by shouting about *der Widerstand* (the Resistance), a German word with which I was familiar, and forced the hapless victim to lie face downwards on a pile of rose clippings. The man's young female colleague, who was now being held immobile by another soldier, watched.

"Frits," Jan whispered after dragging my hand away from his mouth. "The thorns..."

"Shh!" I knew the thorns would hurt the man, but not as much as what I feared was coming.

At a snarled order from the *Zugführer* (commander), the other soldiers began to beat the prisoner with the butts of their rifles. They continued until he was motionless and covered in blood. I didn't see how he could possibly be alive.

Jan tugged my arm, and I turned impatiently. Tears stood in his eyes, but he pointed to the front of his pants, where a dark stain spread from his crotch. I pressed my lips together, shrugged, and kissed his head before continuing to watch.

The *Zugführer* barked another command, and a pair of soldiers hauled the prisoner to his feet, propped him against the nearest tree, and all the soldiers emptied their guns into his back.

Jan gasped. The woman's eyes turned to us, and she quickly dropped to her knees, sobbing loudly. I pulled Jan lower and took the screwdriver out of my pocket, my stomach in my throat. Had they heard him, too?

One of the blood-spattered soldiers spun to face the woman. The *Zugführer* marched over to strike her on the ear before bellowing, "*Schweigen Sie* (be silent)!" right into her face. None of them looked at us. Instead, the soldiers turned, hoisted the man's body up, and flung it onto the rose bushes at the far side of the garden. I was aghast to see a body draped there already.

The wind stopped blowing, the trees ceased rustling, and the moon hid behind the clouds. Jan and I held our breath, and the woman didn't even wipe the spattered blood off her face.

I jumped as raucous laughter split the dark silence before the *Zugführer* pushed the young woman back into the house. His henchmen followed.

My horrified eyes were drawn to the holes in the tree trunk and the shadowy pool of blood at its base. Although that incident might be buried among everything else that happened during World War II, the tree would forever tell the tale.

We remained there, frozen, despite the screams coming from inside the house. Then, realizing that we shouldn't be caught so near to what seemed to be a German base of operations, I pulled Jan to his feet. We returned to *het kindertehuis* via the forest. Only then did I tuck my screwdriver back into my pocket.

Zuster Dermout was angry about how late we were—but not for long. Even that unfeeling woman could see that something beyond words had happened. I curled up in my bed but never told her what. She didn't ask.

It seemed like I'd only just fallen asleep when… "Frits, wake up!"

I sat up with a start, drenched in sweat, my throat on fire. "Wha? I was sleeping, Jan. And it's the middle of the night. What do you want?"

"You were screaming. When I touched you, you tried to punch me!" Jan's voice rose with indignation.

"I'm sorry. I guess it was a nightmare. Next time, leave me be. If you don't touch me while I'm sleeping, I won't hit you."

That was the first of many dreams in which I relived the past.

2

THE BEGINNING

1933 I was born in the year that Hitler became chancellor of Germany, not that I knew it at the time. Nevertheless, that fact would affect my life profoundly. But let me start at the beginning of the story with what my father told me.

Despite the heat having kept her up for most of the night, Mama awoke early on May 3. "Frederik, wake up! It's time."

Papa groaned, pushed away the thin white sheet that had been covering him, and rolled over to peer at his wife. "What is it, *ma chéri*? Are you too hot? Shall I fetch a boy to fan us? Look, the sheet under you is all wet!"

"*Non*, the baby is coming! Help me up."

My 33-year-old Papa's face blanched, and he clutched his dark curls. "Oh, uh…just wait a minute. Stay here…I'll be ready soon." Papa ran around the room, gathering his and her things.

Mama answered through clenched teeth. "Stop dithering. Just go!"

"*Oui, oui*, of course. Sorry." Papa turned to the anxious Congolese houseboy standing at the bedroom door with his face turned toward the hall. "Garçon, get the car started."

After stumbling around while putting on his clothing, Papa helped his 24-year-old wife to the car. It was raining, as was usual in May, so another of their six houseboys held an umbrella over her head. The vehicle bounced over ruts in the dirt road, but eventually, they arrived at the only convent in Léopoldville (now Kinshasa). A missionary nun covered in a long white habit and veil whisked my attractive but distraught mother away. Papa sat down in the hallway to wait, his face buried in his hands.

After several hours, the nun returned. "Monsieur, come meet your son."

"What? A son?" Papa's face broke out in a huge grin, and he hurried to follow the starched lady down the long hallway to the maternity ward.

I'm told that it wasn't hard to find me. I was wailing in a crib by the whitewashed brick wall closest to Mama's bed.

Papa covered the distance to me in three steps and bent over the crib. His warm brown eyes were shining, and his entire body twitched with excitement. "Oh my. He's so little—and very loud. My mother would say he has healthy lungs. I'm so happy I could dance!"

He turned to the nun. "May I pick him up?"

"Of course, he's your child. Just be careful to support his head."

Papa slid his large hands under my head and bottom and carefully lifted me into his arms. Tears of joy sprung from his eyes as he gazed at my face. "Rita, *ma chéri*, you've given me a son! What a gift! I can never thank you enough! Do you want to hold him? Shall I bring him to you?"

My mother raised an elegant hand, her green eyes drooping. "*Non*, I'm tired. You hold him; perhaps take him to another room. He's giving me a headache!"

The normally calm sister gasped audibly.

Papa pressed his lips together, nodded, and handed me to the nun. Pushing his wife's golden-brown hair out of her face, he kissed her forehead. "I understand, *ma chéri*. You must be exhausted. But just so you know, this is how happy I am!"

Papa looped the mosquito net over the bar that hung from the ceiling to encompass the bed. Then he jumped onto my mother's bed and stood on his head, his shirttails flapping around his ears.

Mama's eyes flew open, and she giggled. "Oh, Freddie, I do love you. But, get down. You're embarrassing yourself. And me."

"I told you I would do this if you had a boy. And now I did it." Papa righted himself and took me back from the nun. I was still crying. Bending his face toward me, he gave me my first kiss. My wailing ceased.

"How are you doing, little Frederik?" Papa whispered before turning to Mama. "Shall we give him a middle name? I'd prefer not to, but it's your decision."

"No middle name. I don't like that first name either. It sounds too Catholic, and my father is Jewish. Let's shorten his name to Frits. That seems good to me. What do you think about Frits?"

Papa frowned. "For many generations now, the first son in my family has been Frederik." His eyes softened as he gazed at my face. "But he's very small, so a small name seems appropriate. Fritsje Evenblij. Little Frits. My son. *Oui*, I think that's a fine name."

He lifted me to his face again, and I promptly turned to suck on his cheek.

"Rita, I think our Toni (a French endearment meaning 'beyond praise') is hungry." Papa offered me to my mother.

"Well, I'm sure they have wet nurses here. Ask the sister. Women of my class don't do such things. Now, I really have to sleep." Mama rolled over and presented us with her back.

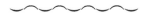

1936   The sheer white curtains blew in the breeze, but the air was stifling. Mama was lounging on a white couch by an open window in our new home in Port Chaltin (now Aketi). As was usual, she wore an elegant outfit with a high neck and tailored skirt, complete with high-heeled shoes. Her hair and nails were perfection. Despite the houseboy fanning her, Mama was shiny with perspiration.

She glanced down at her abdomen, which was again swollen with child, and sighed. Her sullen face betrayed how she felt: she hated living in the Belgian Congo, and she definitely didn't want another baby. Her only hope was that the doctor was right and this child was a girl.

My grandmother always told Mama that men and boys are vastly inferior to women, perhaps because my grandfather abandoned his family when Mama was only a child. Regardless of the reason, Mama constantly repeated what she'd heard her mother say, "Men are only good for waiting on women hand and foot." Taking a sip of palm wine from a cut crystal glass, she grinned to herself. The Congo would absolutely meet with her mother's approval since all the servants were men.

I'd been sitting on the tile floor nearby, arranging ivory and ebony chess pieces in order of their size. Now I grew bored. "Mama, may I go out to play?"

"Yes, please do. Garçon, call Mathieu to watch him."

It amazed me that all our servants had the same last name: Garçon.

"Oui, M'dame." Yohan laid the fan down and turned to me. His eyes creased, and his teeth flashed in an almost blinding smile as he held out his dark brown hand, "Come, Fritsje."

I took his hand after ensuring that all the chess pieces were perfectly in order in their ornately carved box. Together, we skipped to where Mathieu, sitting under a palm tree, was peeling potatoes for dinner. The servants always did both food preparation and cooking outside.

"Call someone else to finish this, Mathieu. Madame would like you to watch Fritsje while I fan her. I think you're his favorite, anyway."

Mathieu crouched down to give me his heart-warming, gap-toothed grin. "Let's find your trike, shall we? Or would you rather go swimming?"

"Swimming, swimming!" I jumped up and down in my excitement.

"Okay, let's get you changed."

Once in my bathing suit, I ran to our private pool, jumping in before Mathieu could catch up. This wasn't as dangerous as it sounds because I'd learned to swim before I could even walk. When I was only a baby, Papa used to throw me into the pool with a tire around my waist. It was the best way to make sure I didn't overheat. Now, I didn't need the tire.

Sweat glistened on Mathieu's forehead as he stood in the shade of a palm tree and watched me splash around. He looked dapper but hot in Papa's shirt, tie, and worn-out woolen suit. Papa gave these to him as part of his wages. Mathieu was the only houseboy to receive a suit, so he didn't complain about the heat. After all, Yohan and the others had to wear their own shorts!

I sent a spray of water in his direction. "Garçon, c...c...come in. Play with me!"

Mathieu glanced over his shoulder before turning back to me. His face was somber. "Fritsje, you know my name. And you also know I'm not allowed in the pool."

I sighed deeply before whining, "Mama isn't watching. And I really, really want you to play. *S'il vous plaît.*"

Shaking his head, Mathieu offered an alternative. "Well, now that you're nice and cool, how about we find your trike? Then I can play with you."

"Oui!" Climbing out of the pool, I threw my wet self into Mathieu's arms. "Carry me!"

Chuckling, Mathieu set my bowl-shaped hat on my head before hoisting me onto his shoulders. I crowed with delight, burying my hands in his wiry curls, heedless of the water running down his jacket. In this fashion, we moved past rows of brightly colored tropical flowers toward the shady side of our property.

"There it is! It's red, you know!" I began to slide off Mathieu's shoulders.

"Hey, be careful there. I'm pretty sure I'm not allowed to drop you!"

I giggled. "You won't do that because you love me. Just like P…P…Papa does."

Clearing his throat, Mathieu nodded. "Okay then, let's race. You cycle to that tree, and I'll run. Ready, set, go!"

We played this game, where I won the majority of "races" for an hour.

"Okay, Fritsje, now it's time for me to assist with preparing the meal."

"Can I help?"

Mathieu ruffled my blond curls before stroking my cheek. "I was hoping you'd offer, Fritsje Evenblij. That'd be great!"

I grabbed his hand and held it there. "I love you, Mathieu Garçon."

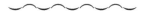

Mama had been gone for several days, leaving me in the care of "the boys." I didn't see Papa except at bedtime, but that was normal. Papa needed to work at the Nieuwe Afrikaanse Handels-Vennootschap (NAHV), a company helping build the Cape Town to Cairo railway. He was an accountant, which Papa told me meant he counted money.

Therefore, it was a surprise when he entered my bedroom during my afternoon nap. "Toni, wake up. There's someone I want you to meet." He picked me up and carried me in his muscular arms into Mama's frilly pink and white bedroom. She was reclining on the bed and dressed in a silky white nightdress.

My forehead wrinkled. It was daytime. Why wasn't Mama on the chaise lounge in the living room? I had just opened my mouth to ask when I heard a reedy wail coming from a little bassinet in the room's corner. The volume of the cries increased.

I pointed wordlessly. Papa carried me over to the cot and pushed aside the mosquito net. There, lying on his back, was a now red-faced infant, screaming for all he was worth. I thought he resembled one of the monkeys that frequented our trees.

I recoiled in shock. "Who's that? Why's it here?"

Papa chuckled, put me down, and gently picked the baby up. His shock of blond hair stood up like a brush. "This is your brother, Jan."

"Um, Papa," I whispered. "He's kind of loud and ugly. Mama prob'ly won't like him. M..m...maybe we should give him back."

Truth be told, if that had been possible, Mama would probably have done it. I later learned that, upon seeing her new baby was a boy, she'd sworn in a most unladylike manner and burst into floods of tears.

Now, to my astonishment, Papa had a quite different reaction. He threw his head back and roared with laughter. "There'll be no giving back, Toni. He's ours. And you're his big brother. Do you know what that means?"

I backed away, put my thumb in my mouth, and mumbled around it. "What?"

"Come here."

Being rocked by his loving father, Jan stopped squalling, so I cautiously drew nearer. Maybe the monkey look-alike wasn't so bad. I stretched out one hopeful but grimy finger. "Can I touch him?"

"Of course, but be gentle and only touch his cheek or hands."

I carefully stroked my new brother's soft cheek while Papa continued. "From now on, our Jan is *ton petit frère* (your little brother in French). Let's call him Jean-Jean. It'll take time, but one day, he'll be your friend, too. You'll teach Jean-Jean all the important things, like how to ride a red tricycle and throw a ball."

I frowned. "Papa, his legs won't reach the pedals. He's too little."

Papa's eyes sparkled. "He'll grow. And you'll need to protect him while he does. Do you understand?"

The weight of this responsibility would eventually round my shoulders, but I nodded wordlessly. I would have promised anything to please my father.

Mama raised herself up on one elbow. "Freddie, I've done my duty to you now. You know I never wanted children, especially sons. But here we are. I'm thrilled for you, but please take the boys out now. It's so hot, and I'm so tired; I need to sleep."

Papa sighed. "Come on, Toni."

Carefully cradling my brother, he led me from the room, but it was too late. I'd heard what Mama said. Could it be true? Didn't she want my baby brother and me? Didn't she love us? I turned toward Papa to ask him, but he was engrossed in gazing at his new son.

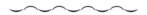

1937 "Papa, you're home!" I threw myself into my father's arms.

With a smile lighting his face, Papa returned my embrace before lifting me up, sitting in his favorite chair, and settling me on his lap. "Tell me. What has my Toni been doing today?"

"I swam and swam and even helped Mathieu throw Jean-Jean into the pool." I hesitated before wrinkling my nose. "He really, really didn't like it."

"How do you know? What happened?"

"He screamed and screamed. And Mama came outside and said, 'Garçon, stop him from making that infernal noise!' Papa, what does 'infernal' mean? Why did she say that? Why?"

"It means 'terrible.' So, did he?"

"Yes, Mathieu hooked my long stick into the tire around Jean-Jean. Then he pulled him to the side of the pool. After he got him out, I told Mathieu never to throw Jean-Jean in again. I protected him, right?" I leaned back to bask in the approval I was sure I'd see in my father's face.

"Yes, you did. Well done. But Papa thinks it's okay to let the boys put Jean-Jean in the pool, don't you?"

"I guess so." I put my head on one side. "Why?"

"Because it's so hot here, and *ton petit frère* needs to learn to swim. Maybe you could teach him."

"Yeah, maybe I could. And you know what else? I stepped in an enormous pile of elephant poo. It was right after Mathieu showed me a great big snake. The poo went to my knees! But it's a secret. Mathieu said Mama wouldn't be happy about the p...p...poo. Or the snake..."

Papa chuckled. "Oh my! I thought there was a smell in here."

I frowned and bent over to inspect my browned legs. "He washed me before I went in the pool. Did he miss some?"

"*Non, non,* Papa was just teasing. You smell fine." Papa drew me closer, yawned, and closed one eye.

"Um, Papa...is there a fly in your eye?" I screwed up my eyes, trying to copy what he was doing.

11

"*Non,* that eye just seems to be tired."

"But why's only one eye tired? Why?"

"I can't answer all your questions right now, Fritsje. I think all of me is tired. Go on. Let Papa close his eyes for a while."

Feeling a little anxious at this strange behavior from Papa, I slid down from his lap and went outside. He was usually never too tired to answer my endless questions. Maybe I could help one of the houseboys to make dinner.

Over the next few months, I noticed Papa winking at me more often. He also sometimes struggled with picking his knife and fork up at dinner. Polite eating was essential in our family, so it was shocking when he occasionally gave up and ate with his fingers.

Mama covered her husband's trembling hand. "Freddie, Freddie, what's going on? You're so tired these days. I'm worried. You need to see *un docteur.*"

"You're right. I thought I was just exhausted from this terrible climate. There's no escaping the heat and humidity! But it's gone too far. I'll go as soon as I can."

Only a week later, Papa came home with rounded shoulders. He spoke in a low voice. "Rita, could you ask one of the boys to make us a drink, and then let's sit down. I have news."

He continued once they were seated, and Jan was on Papa's lap. "I went to *le docteur.* He says it's not malaria or sleeping sickness. Frankly, he has no idea what's wrong with me—except that he thinks it might be serious."

Mama covered her mouth as her eyes grew round. Glancing between my parents' unhappy faces, it felt like time stopped, and I moved to slip my hand into my father's.

"He advised me to go to the Netherlands, where they have more equipment and better hospitals. We're due a sabbatical anyway, but it looks like now it'll happen sooner rather than later."

My ears pricked up. I knew from what Papa had told me I'd been to the Netherlands before, but I didn't remember it. Now, it seemed we would go again. What an adventure!

Interrupting was strictly forbidden, but I did it anyway, my hands dancing and twirling with excitement. "Will we go on a b…b…boat again?"

Papa answered, "*Non,* I think this time we'll fly. Jean-Jean is too young, and I'm too tired to handle the long journey. It's over 10,000 kilometers by sea!"

"Fly? *Non,* you're being silly. We don't have wings!" I put my arms out and zoomed around the room before screeching to a halt in front of Papa.

"How would you like to fly in an airplane, Fritsje? Just like a bird in the sky." He turned to Mama. "The company said they'd pay for that this time."

I opened my mouth to ask more, but Mama frowned at me before joining the conversation again. "That's so good to hear. I'm certainly looking forward to a break from this infernal weather. And we can show Jean-Jean to my mother and your family."

She stared into space before again focusing on Papa. "And perhaps we can get some answers about you, my Freddie."

"Infernal," I whispered under my breath.

"Frits…" came the warning, and I was silent.

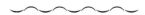

"Guess what, Mathieu! We're going on an airplane. Have you ever been on one?" I was again trembling with excitement, my hands twirling of their own volition.

"*Non,* I never have."

"What about you, Yohan?"

"Me neither."

"Why not? Aren't boys allowed on airplanes? Why?" I knew there were all kinds of places our houseboys weren't allowed to go. They weren't even permitted to sit on the same benches as us! Was this another one of those inexplicable rules?

Just then, my mother's voice came floating out. "Garçon, Jean-Jean is awake. Please get him up and give him his lunch." Mama always insisted that we be kept as far away from her as possible, preferably at the end of the porch between the servant's quarters.

Both men hurried away, perhaps relieved not to have to answer my questions or maybe just aware that there was much to do.

Over the following weeks, the houseboys hand-washed our clothes and packed our suitcases. They also washed our bedding and the curtains, scrubbed the floors, and flung covers over the furniture. I tried to assist, but Yohan told me I was more helpful as an overseer. That meant I got to sit on a chair and watch.

Gazing around the room while bouncing up and down on my chair, my questions again overflowed. "Yohan, how many nights sleeping until we get back? What will you do while we're gone? Will you take care of my tricycle? Can you carve more animals?" I had an impressive collection of hand-carved jungle animals on the shelf in my bedroom.

Yohan wiped the sweat from his forehead before answering. "You'll be gone for six months, which is over 100 nights sleeping. That'll allow me to spend more time with my wife and children. But of course, I'll take special care of your trike. As for carving animals, I only do that for good boys."

My face fell. "I'm not good. Mama says I'm loud and rambunctious. What's rambunctious, Yohan?"

"It means you're exactly the way you should be. So, I think there will be carved animals waiting when you get back."

I scowled, pretty sure that this wasn't what Mama meant, but so glad Yohan didn't know. I could always count on the boys to think I was wonderful.

"Could you give me earrings like yours?" I reached up to put my finger through the gleaming gold.

Yohan chuckled, "Go and play, you scamp!"

The day finally arrived. Mathieu dressed me in a white shirt, white knee socks, white woolen shorts, and a blue jacket. "Mama, this jacket is so hot! Can I take it off?"

"*Non*. Stop complaining, Fritsje. You'll be very glad you have it when we arrive. Now, it's time we went."

I looked at her in surprise. What could she mean? Why would anyone ever need to wear so many layers?

"Get in the car, Frits." Papa bent to hand Jean-Jean to Mama.

Suddenly, my eyes grew round and filled with tears. "Matthieu! Yohan! Where are they? I need a good-bye kiss!"

Mama groaned. "Put him in the car, Freddie. There'll be no houseboy kisses."

I sobbed all the way to the airport.

Papa working at the Niewe Afrikansche Handels-Venootschap, Belgian Congo, 1933. (top)

Frits and an unnamed houseboy in Léopoldville, Belgian Congo, 1934. (bottom)

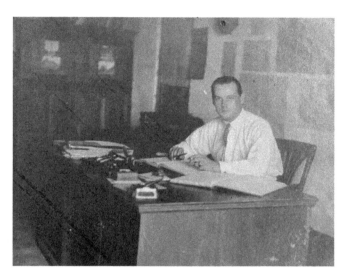

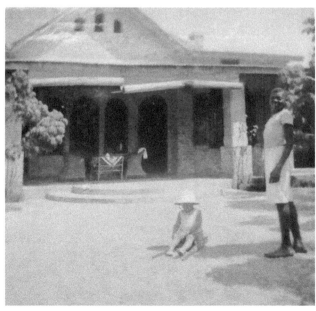

Mama with Frits and Jan in Aketi, Belgian Congo, 1937.

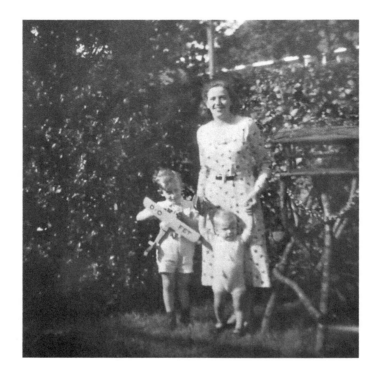

3

THE MOVE

1938 In January, my family and I traveled to Schiphol Airport in the Netherlands on a Sabena Airlines flight. Papa was wearing a suit; Mama was in an elegant dress, hat, and high heels; and Jan and I wore our itchy clothing and very peculiar hats.

Mama sighed and shook her head as we stood up and stretched our legs upon landing. "Frits, even when you've been doing nothing, you manage to look totally disheveled, like a bag of rags." She quickly tucked in my shirt and, after spitting on her handkerchief, wiped my mouth.

As soon as I could escape Mama's clutches, I sprinted down the aisle to the airplane exit, where steep metal stairs had been lowered from the door. What was this place like? Papa said there wouldn't be any monkeys or elephants. What would be there instead? I could hardly wait to find out.

I stopped in shock at the door. How strange! It was 90°F and sunny when we took off, but now it was 34°F and nearly dark. Even the rain was icy! I hoped it wouldn't always be like this.

"Come on, Fritsje. Help Papa down these stairs."

Puffing up my chest, I carefully held both the railing and my father's hand. Mama, holding Jan's, followed.

"Papa, where are the boys? Who will drive us to Oma's (grandmother's) house?"

"We'll take a taxi. See, they're over there!" Papa put his fingers to his lips and emitted a shrill whistle.

I pressed my nose to the window of the black taxi and felt my entire body stiffen with excitement. My hands and feet were twirling as I once again felt questions bubbling up. "Papa, we're going so fast!

Everything is blurred. Where are the palm trees? Ooo, the trees have no leaves. They're naked! Where are the leaves? Where are the pretty plants? Look at that water-road! Why…"

"Stop right there, Frits. Let your father rest. We're much too tired to answer your endless questions." Mama's voice cut like glass. "And *doe maar gewoon* (just act normal)!"

"But I want to know! Why do they put water in roads? What's Oma's house like? Does she have a pool? Does she have a red t…t…tricycle?"

Papa turned to give me one of those looks. I fell silent.

The taxi finally stopped outside a red brick house in Den Haag (The Hague). I was utterly astonished to see that the narrow-bricked road joined the sidewalk, out of which the tall row houses ascended almost to the sky. The only place one could see plants was in the window boxes.

"Papa, why are the houses all stuck together? Why…"

He shook his head at me just before Mama rang the brass doorbell in front of us. The door swung open. There stood a statuesque gray-haired lady in a dark dress with a lacey shawl. I scrunched up my nose; she smelled strongly of perfume. I preferred the smell of the jungle. Or even of elephant poo.

"Ah, you're all here. Come in quick before you're completely soaked. I'll make some nice hot tea," my grandmother said.

"*Goedemiddag,* Oma," I said in carefully rehearsed Dutch.

"Don't call me 'Oma.' It makes me feel old. I'm Tante Aleida."

My eyes grew round as I gazed at her wrinkled face. Didn't she know she was old?

"Go on, *mon petit enfant* (my little child). Don't be shy." Papa gave me a little push from behind. Tante Aleida led the way into the living room, closely followed by Mama.

I gazed around the small room, which was crowded with furniture. Everything looked so heavy, from the dark blue velvet curtains and the blue patterned rug to the wooden cabinet and plush sofa. My eyes lit on a rectangular, black metal chair-sized thing that seemed to glow from within. What was that? I pointed wordlessly.

Papa knelt and enclosed me in his arm. "That's the *kachel* (coal-burning stove). All Dutch houses have one; it keeps them warm. But don't touch it. Papa doesn't want you to burn your hand."

I nodded and pressed my little body closer to him. "Um, Papa, where is my grand-père? I only see Tante Aleida. She doesn't like me," I whispered in French. I was more curious than worried about this. In

18

my albeit limited experience, men were always more affectionate than women.

Mama turned, also speaking French. "Frits, I told you. My father, your grandfather, lives in Indonesia."

My eyes grew round. "Why? What's he doing there?"

"He's a Vaudeville artist, an entertainer." Mama's mouth twisted before she added under her breath, "And he gallivants with women."

Tante Aleida gasped, but I didn't notice, having heard but unsure what Mama meant. "What's Vaudeville? What's gallivant? I want to gallivant!"

"Rita!" came the warning from Papa before he silenced me with a look.

Seeing that I wasn't going to get an answer to my questions, I turned my attention to the big and little tables in the living room. The big table had a plate of cookies, delicate side plates with a floral pattern, matching cups and saucers, and a teapot. The small one also had side plates, cups, and saucers, but they were more robust.

"Frits, you and Jan sit over there at the little table. You may each have *één speculaasje* (one spice cookie). I'll pour you some lemonade. Be careful not to spill."

"*Dank u wel* (thank you), Tante Aleida," I answered in Dutch as I'd been taught before turning and speaking French to my father. "Papa, why is she pouring my lemonade? Where are her boys? Are they gallivanting?"

Papa silenced me with a look, then pulled out a chair for my mother to take a seat at the bigger table. She carefully placed the napkin on her lap. "Thank you so much for agreeing to have us until we can move into our apartment. How have you been, Mama?"

The adults continued to talk and sip their tea, and Jan and I each finished our cookie and drink. Growing restless, I slipped off my chair to explore. My eyes lit up when I spotted a chess set. "Look, Jean-Jean," I whispered. "This one is the k…k…king; this one is the queen; these are the horses, and these are the castles."

Jan, squatting in the way of all babies, mutely pointed at the remaining pieces before popping one in his mouth.

"Jean-Jean, *non*!" I hauled the peon out. "These are the people. You can't eat them. Let's line them up so they can go for a walk."

"Frits, Jan! What are you doing? Did I say you could get down from the table?"

"Rita, *ma chéri*, they're very young and have been cooped up too long. I'll take them for a walk." Papa stood up from his chair and promptly fell over.

I stood frozen in shock. What was Papa doing? I was sure Tante Aleida wouldn't like this game.

"Freddie!" Mama jumped up. "What happened? Are you hurt?"

"*Non*, I think I'm just tired. Moeder, please show me to our room. I need to lie down."

As Tante Aleida and Mama helped Papa to his bed, I turned to Jean-Jean, who was staring after Papa with his fingers in his mouth. "Don't worry, Jean-Jean. Papa will be okay after he sleeps. Now, help me clean up."

As I guided his little fingers to place the chess pieces back in the box, keeping a close eye that none of them ended up in his mouth, I reflected on what I'd told him. The trouble was that I wasn't sure I was telling my brother the truth.

~~~~~~~

Papa bent over my bed. "Wake up, sleepyhead. Today, we'll move into our very own Netherlands apartment on the Haringkade."

The net curtains billowed as an artic blast blew through the open window. I shivered and slid deeper under the rather itchy covers. "Will it be warm? Will the boys be there? Will I have a red tricycle?"

Hauling me out of bed, Papa chuckled as he helped me into my woolen clothing. "Oh, Toni, this country is cold everywhere. But the apartment has a lovely *kachel* where we can warm your clothes before you put them on. As for houseboys, *non,* we won't have those. We can only afford one servant, so you'll have to be a helper."

My forehead wrinkled. "But Papa, I don't know how to clean. And I'm not allowed to touch the firepit and cook."

"Hush, *mon petit enfant.* Papa knows you'll be able to do everything you'll need to do. You're clever and strong and kind. You can do it."

"The boys said I'm a good helper…"

After patting my curly head, Papa laboriously hauled himself to his feet and turned to the crib. Jan was standing in his flannel pajamas, babbling something incomprehensible. "Okay, I hear you, *doux bébé* (sweet baby). Come to Papa."

After a breakfast of milk, brown bread, Edam cheese, and my favorite boiled eggs, Mama air-kissed Tante Aleida goodbye on both her cheeks. Papa did the same, then indicated with his head that I should follow suit. Not a chance! I put my hands behind my back, set my jaw, and looked at my feet. I genuinely did not want to touch, let alone kiss, those wrinkled cheeks.

"Frits!" came the warning from Mama.

"*Non,*" I screamed, surprising even myself with my rage. "I don't want to kiss Tante Aleida. I don't like her!"

My grandmother inhaled audibly, her chest swelling up to a truly impressive size. Mama went pale. Papa's lips were white as he grabbed my arm and swatted my backside. "Say you're sorry!"

"*Non, non, non!* I'm not sorry. Her face is ugly. And she's stinky. And I'll never do it. And…"

Then I glimpsed Papa's face, and tears began to roll down my cheeks. "I want to go hooome!"

Mama folded her arms while Papa bent down to take me into his. "Toni, this won't work. Say you're sorry and kiss her."

By now hiccupping my sobs, I looked at my feet while mumbling, "*Je suis désolé*, Tante Aleida." I peeked up to see if that was enough. Apparently not.

The patrician matriarch smiled grimly, pointed to her cheek, and bent down to my level. I glanced at Papa. Could he mean it? Apparently, yes. So, very reluctantly, I did my duty before flinging myself at Papa's legs. To my astonishment, he nearly fell over again, catching himself on a nearby chest. Was I that strong?

"As soon as we're settled, Freddie." Mama's voice boded no argument.

After a taxi ride where we left the brick jungle of the city and passed by the trees and greenery of the street called the Scheveningseweg, we came to our new home. I gazed out the car's back window at the trees and meadows. Today, the sky was a bright blue, even if the wind was howling. Maybe this wouldn't be so bad after all. Especially if we didn't have to live with Tante Aleida! I hoped that, inside at least, our home would look a lot like the house in Aketi.

Mama carried Jan while Papa held my hand and paid for the taxi. Digging a key out of his pocket, he unlocked and pushed the apartment door open.

My blue eyes grew round. Unlike our home in the Congo, which was white with big, airy rooms, the door here opened onto a dark, steep staircase. Leaving my family behind, I scrambled to the top, screeching

21

to a halt in front of a tiny indoor kitchen with a tile countertop and running water. How strange to have the kitchen indoors! I figured probably the firepit would be on the balcony that I could see through the kitchen window, but even standing on my toes, wasn't tall enough to check.

I turned slowly. The living room was similar to Tante Aleida's, being furnished with carved wooden cabinets, a chaise lounge, a sofa, and an easy chair, this time all in red velvet. The floor, dining, and side tables were covered in rugs! Could it be that Dutch people also walked on their tables? I thought that might be fun.

There was one other door on that floor, and I opened it curiously to find that it contained an indoor toilet and a tiny sink, just like at my grandmother's. I sniffed cautiously. It didn't stink, unlike our outhouse in the Congo. And, like at Tante Aleida's house, there was water in the bottom of the toilet! But here she wasn't watching... I was just going to reach down and touch the water when Mama's shriek made me pull my hand back. "Frits, you must never touch toilet water. Never. It's dirty!"

Strange. It looked clean to me. I shrugged.

There was something (or someone) missing—a pair of "someones" who'd always made my house a home. They were probably busy upstairs. I darted through a door in the living room and up the next flight of stairs but only found two bedrooms. One had two small beds with crisp white sheets and heavy woolen blankets. The other had a double bed and a wooden dresser with a mirror perfect for watching myself pull faces. Later.

Frowning, I raced back down the stairs and planted myself in front of Papa. "Where are the boys?"

"No, boys, Toni. I told you. Remember? We'll have a servant, but only one, and Mademoiselle Marijke won't sleep here. You'll have to do some chores."

I remembered him telling me that before, but it sounded no better now than it did then. Tears sprung to my eyes, and I stamped my foot. "I don't like this place. I don't want a *mademoiselle*. I want the b...b...boys! I want to go home!"

Papa quickly led me to the front window. "But look, Fritsje, can you see the ocean there? You can watch the waves and the boats any time you want. And, you know what else? This place is near a park where you can walk through trees and flower gardens and chase geese."

"By myself?" I sucked in a big breath.

"Well, you're a very big boy, almost grown up, but I think Papa will go with you. Since he won't be going to work, he'll have lots of time. It's going to be wonderful! You'll see."

Finally, we were unpacked. I pretty soon learned we weren't allowed to walk on the tables and that the rug was removed from the big table before we ate. Mama would replace it with a pristine white tablecloth, and Heaven help us if we got it dirty. With no boys, Mademoiselle Marijke had to take everything to the laundry service. Mama made it known that women of her class didn't do those things. I wondered what they did do but knew enough not to ask.

We'd been in our home for about a week when the doorbell rang just after our dinner of *hutspot* (mashed potatoes, carrots, and onions) and gravy.

"Fritsje, I'm busy making coffee. Open the door," said Mama.

Jan was playing at Mama's feet with a bowl and wooden spoon, but he was too little to open doors. And Mademoiselle Marijke was washing the dishes.

The problem was that I was also otherwise engaged. Being focused on turning a piece of glass this way and that, to see how the light from a nearby lamp would be refracted or reflected by the angle of the glass, I didn't even bother to answer Mama.

"Frits, now!" Papa's voice was stern.

Oops! I ran to pull on the rope that was connected to the doorknob at the bottom of the stairs. Papa had shown me earlier how it worked.

I watched as, almost miraculously, the door opened, admitting an arctic blast of wind. At the bottom of the stairs, an elderly gentleman wearing a stylish black coat and carrying an umbrella smiled up at me.

"*Goedenavond, jongeman* (Good evening, young man). Is your father home?"

"Papa," I called over my shoulder. "There's an old man here to see you."

I heard Mama inhale from the kitchen and braced myself for another inexplicable explosion, but Papa interrupted just in time.

"It's *le docteur*. Invite him in." Papa, who was often exhausted, was sitting in his favorite chair watching the unending, seemingly

23

horizontal rain streak the window. This phenomenon also fascinated me: the rain in the Congo, while plentiful, always fell downwards.

I did as I was told, proudly speaking some of the little carefully enunciated Dutch I'd picked up. The bespectacled man ascended the stairs before handing me his heavy coat. I couldn't reach the coat rack, so dropped it on the floor, my eye caught by the gold pocket watch gleaming against his brown suit. Clearly, this was a man in charge of his life.

"Dokter Smit, thank you so much for coming." Mama emerged from the kitchen, running her hands over her always smooth hair. She picked up the coat with a frown at me. "Meneer Evenblij is through here. Would you like some coffee?" Then, under her breath to remind me of my manners, she murmured, "Frits!"

Coming to myself with a start, I closed my mouth before carefully placing the doctor's umbrella in the stand at the top of the stairs. Then, knowing full well that I shouldn't, I slid down the wall just outside the living room. This might be my chance to find out what was wrong with Papa.

After Marijke took the coffee through, Dokter Smit pulled a chair up next to Papa and put his stethoscope in his ears. Mama, seeing me, closed the door and shut me out. Now, even with my ear pressed to the wooden door, much to Marijke's amusement, I could only hear murmurs.

It seemed like hours later when I heard footsteps approaching the living room door. Jumping up, I casually strolled into the kitchen. As the door opened, I heard the doctor's voice but had little idea what he was saying.

"Meneer Evenblij, your muscles seem far too weak to me. I'm uncertain of the cause, so recommend that you go to the medical facility in Leiden. They have the right equipment to do the necessary testing. They'll stimulate your nerves repetitively; the muscle response should tell us more."

Papa was admitted to the hospital in Leiden almost immediately. He was only there for a few days, but getting the results took longer. Over the next month, Papa was often distracted. Sometimes, he was tearful. I didn't understand what was happening but found that Papa seemed calmer if I perched on his lap and stroked his hair. Eventually, the physicians in Leiden mailed their findings to Dokter Smit. He came to our house again.

Seated next to Papa, the elderly gentleman spoke kindly. "I'm so sorry, but I have bad news." I understood that and felt a chill go through my body.

The doctor continued, "The physicians in Leiden are sure you have myasthenia gravis. It's an incurable disease, and the prognosis isn't good. I'm expecting that in a couple of years, you'll no longer be able to walk."

Papa jerked as if someone hit him. "What? I thought I heard you say…"

Mama's back remained ramrod straight, but her voice trembled. "Is there a treatment, dokter?"

Dokter Smit leaned forward and took her hand in both of his. "Yes, but it's not great. We can give neostigmine, but that drug has lots of very unpleasant side effects. Well, if we can get it, given the situation in Germany." Mama pulled her hand out of the doctor's. "And you, sir, will need to rest," he continued.

Papa took a deep breath, squared his shoulders, and raised his chin. "Well, there are worse things than not being able to walk. I can work sitting on a chair. That's what I do, anyway!"

I stood motionless, barely breathing, wondering why the doctor continued to look so solemn, even though Papa seemed to think things were okay.

Papa beckoned me to his side and enclosed me in the circle of his arm. I leaned my head on him and inhaled the fragrance that brought me peace. The smell of my father: sandalwood shaving foam, newsprint, cigars, and just him.

"Thank you for letting us know, dokter. We'll do the best we can." A nod from Mama signaled to Mademoiselle Marijke that she should take Dokter Smit's coat off the rack and help him put it on.

The doctor continued speaking while he did up the buttons and adjusted his scarf. "Meneer Evenblij, I want to get you into the hospital next week so we can begin a course of treatment. Maybe we can delay the inevitable."

Papa nodded silently, just as the clock chimed four.

"*Bedankt* (thanks), Dokter Smit." Mama watched until the door closed before throwing herself down on the chaise lounge and putting her hand against her forehead. "Marijke, please bring me a glass of wine. I need one."

I glanced up at Papa. After having risen to his feet to bid the doctor farewell, he was pale and trembling. "Sit down, Papa. I'll help Marijke get you one, too. I'm very careful."

Papa rubbed my head when I set the wine beside him without spilling a drop, giving me what was becoming a familiar wink. "Thank you, Toni. You're such a good boy. Quite beyond praise."

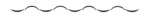

The sun was shining through my window when Jan climbed into my bed. "Well, *bonjour*!" I chuckled. "Looks like it's time to get dressed. Let's surprise Mama—I'll help you."

Unfortunately, wriggling a squirmy toddler into clothes wasn't as easy as I'd assumed. "Jean-Jean, keep still!"

Just then, I heard Papa's cheerful whistle outside our room. "Papa, I need help!"

Immediately, the door opened. "Happy Birthday, Toni! You're five now. A big boy! What did you need help with...oh!" Papa's voice slowed as he took in my situation. "You're a big boy, but Papa thinks you should leave dressing two-year-olds at least until you're six. Now, come to Papa, *doux bébé.*"

As Papa completed the challenging job, I quickly put on my clothes before running to the kitchen. There, I washed my hands three times and my face once before noticing a heavenly smell. There was a beautiful chocolate cake on the counter! Were we going to have visitors? My body stiffened, and my hands began dancing. I quickly tucked them under my arms. Mama had told me, "*doe maar gewoon*" too many times for me to forget, and I knew big boys don't twirl their hands!

"Oh, there you are, Fritsje." Mama entered the kitchen with a rustle of skirts and her usual cloud of French perfume. Papa always told me that my mother was a beautiful woman, but as I stood staring, deep in thought, she still just looked like Mama: cool, elegant, unsmiling.

"Happy Birthday! Today, we're going to have such a special day. Tante Aleida, Tante Roo (my father's mother), Opa (my grandpa and father's father), and many other relatives are coming to celebrate that you're five. That's the tradition here in the Netherlands, you know." She paused before narrowing her eyes. "Since you're a big boy now, you'd better behave."

My heart began to race. "Mama, please, I want to play with the magnet Papa gave me. May I stay in my room while they're here? I could take care of Jan. I don't even need any cake." That last offer should clinch the deal!

"Nonsense! That would be rude. Refined people don't behave like that. It's your day, and you'll have to be the host."

"But I don't want to." My voice grew louder as I realized the inevitability of what would happen. "I won't. *Non!* You can't make me." I tried to run away, but Mama was faster.

Grabbing me by the arm, she exerted pressure with her perfectly manicured nails and spoke through clenched teeth. "I can, and you will."

Just then, Papa came down the stairs, Jean-Jean in his arms. "What's all this noise Papa hears, Toni?"

By now, cold sweat had gathered on my neck, and tears were streaming down my face. "Papa, people are coming, and I don't like it. I don't want to see stinky Tante Aleida and Tante Roo. D…d…don't make me!"

Papa knelt on the floor, put Jan down, and gathered me close to his heart. "Toni, I know it seems scary, but everyone will be here to celebrate your birthday. They'll all say, '*Hartelijk gefeliciteerd met je verjaardag* (Happy Birthday in Dutch)' to you, me, Mama, and Jean-Jean! Then, you'll have a piece of yummy cake and some sparkling lemonade. And, because you're the birthday boy, you can eat while sitting on my lap."

That was a very rare thing indeed, and I took a deep breath. "Really, Papa?"

Mama made a noise. After giving her a look, Papa nodded. "I promise."

So, I spent the afternoon perched in my favorite place, comparing how my magnet stuck to a spoon, a nail, and a pen. Whenever someone new came up the stairs, I buried my face in Papa's chest and refused to look at them. Mama murmured in French about manners, but Papa was my protector. And I could still eat chocolate cake. That made it all okay.

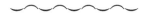

In August of 1938, while dahlias were filling the Netherlands with joy, Papa greeted Mama with a long face. "Rita, come sit down next to me. I have bad news."

"What could be worse than the news we've had?" Mama, who'd just returned from visiting Tante Aleida, moved Jan from the couch to the floor and settled herself next to Papa. Papa was speaking in a monotone that was most unlike him. I continued working on my puzzle but listened carefully to what my parents were saying.

"Well, with our sabbatical months being over, my boss asked when we would return to the Congo. I'm afraid I had to tell him it won't be for a while. After all, I still need medical treatment. He asked why the delay and I had no choice but to tell him about my diagnosis. He didn't fire me but said he had no choice but to reduce me to sick pay only."

Mama gasped and pressed her fist to her mouth. "Oh, Freddie! What will we live on? We can't eat air! Where will we live? The rent here…"

Papa's eyes became red, and a tear overflowed. "I saved up a bit, so with my sick pay and help from the government, we can afford our rent for a year. But not much more. I don't know what else to do…"

Mama took a deep breath, her nostrils flaring. "It looks like now I'll have to be the provider for this family. Who knows how long we'll have to stay here?"

My throat felt tight as panic overwhelmed me. Would we have to live in this cold, unwelcoming place forever? "Papa, *non*! I want to go home! I don't like stupid yucky Den Haag!" I jumped to my feet and sobbed loudly, causing Jan to follow suit.

"Stop that noise right now!" Mama stood and drew herself up to her full height. "No sniveling. That won't help. It never has, and it never will. You might as well learn now."

Papa's shoulders were rounded, but he pulled Jan onto his lap and drew me to his side. "I wish I knew what to do, Mommy." His voice broke, but he still held me tight.

Mama turned on him. "I'm not your 'mommy,' and you can't do anything. It's up to me. I'm an intelligent and capable woman. I'll get a job and support you and your children."

Papa opened his mouth to speak, but Mama continued spitting out her plans. "We'll see if De Viersprong, *het kindertehuis* in Driebergen, will take the children at short notice. Mama recommended that place as somewhere where high-minded people would raise our boys. It'll be for the best. After all, we were going to leave them there when we returned to the Congo anyway…"

My eyes bulged, and my mouth dropped as the suspicion that Mama honestly didn't want us seemed to be confirmed through her words.

"I wish I could…" Papa's voice broke.

"But you can't." Mama narrowed her eyes. "And you can stop your sniveling, too."

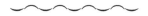

About a week later, Mama came home with what she said was good news. "Freddie, I found a job! It wasn't easy with the economy as it is, but I'll be doing office work. You know how I enjoy writing—this is the next best thing."

Papa struggled to stand up from the chair that was becoming a part of his body. "That's great news, Mommy. Where?"

"It's here in Den Haag, and when we need it, the job comes with a room I can rent. The pay is pretty bad, but it's better than nothing. I accepted the offer." Mama busied herself, pulling off her gloves and hanging up her coat before tidying her hair in the mirror.

"But I'll be spending time in Leiden. It's so far…"

"We need to do what we have to do. You're already barely able to manage. The nurses at *het kindertehuis* said that they can take the boys in October, so I'll be free to focus on work. You can live with your sister when you're not in the hospital. We might even be able to afford to get you a part-time nurse."

Papa's face fell. "Rita, Jean-Jean is still little, only two. And Toni needs so much special attention. I crave having the boys close by. Couldn't we all somehow stay together? Maybe your mother could help."

"*Non*, I already asked her. She doesn't want to. You know she doesn't like children. And I can't send the boys just anywhere because I don't want them to be raised by a working-class person."

"I hate this! It's terrible!" Papa put his face in his trembling hands.

"Well, we've known for some time that it's inevitable. There's no use crying. It can't be helped."

"How much does having the boys board cost? Do we have enough?" Papa appeared to be grasping at straws, and I hoped he'd catch one.

"That's also good news. It's a marvelous place—unfortunately, more than we can afford now, but the nurses at *het kindertehuis* will work with us. They said Frits can earn part of his and Jan's keep by doing extra chores." Mama gave me one of her looks. "Maybe they'll discipline him enough so he becomes less difficult."

"Non, ma chéri! Toni's only a child! And he can't help how he is. I'm not happy about this at all." Papa stared down at his hands.

Mama put her hand on her hip. "Well then, you come up with a better plan. And since you won't, I'll start the job on Monday."

"Hopefully, when you and the boys aren't living with me, I can still see you all sometimes." Papa's voice became high with emotion.

Examining a radio that Papa had helped me take apart distracted me during some of this conversation. But now, alarm bells began to ring in my head. My stomach clenched, I began to vibrate, and the inevitable happened: the volcano erupted.

"Noooo!" I screamed. "I want to stay with Papa, not with stinky Tante Aleida, and not with some stupid nurses!" I threw the radio to the floor, causing it to shatter into almost as many pieces as my heart.

Mama, doubtless thinking that the nurses would never accept me if I had a tantrum as soon as I arrived, crouched down. "Fritsje, Papa is going to the hospital in Leiden, then to a rest home, and then to your aunt's house. That wouldn't be much fun for you. The home in Driebergen won't be so bad. Jean-Jean is going, too, so you can help take care of him. There'll be lots of toys and magnets, and probably more electric things that you can take apart. Also, the nice nurses told me that every day during the summer, they take the children to a lake where they can swim! They call it a pool."

A lake that's called a pool! That captured my imagination. Wiping my nose on my sleeve, earning a groan from Mama, I quietened down to listen.

Mama looked up at Papa. "And, best of all, the home is near a forest with ponds in it. You'll probably get to play there all the time."

"B…b…but, I want Papa…"

Papa lifted me onto his lap. "And Papa wants you, my Toni. But I'm sick and need to rest, so I'll get better. We have no choice. You'll need to be Papa's good big boy. I'll be depending on you to take care of Jean-Jean."

"I love you, Papa," I murmured as I listened to the rhythmic beat of his heart and enjoyed his fragrance while resting my head on his chest.

The thought of leaving my precious Papa was more than my young psyche could handle, so I soon slipped off his lap to examine the pieces of the radio. Just how did it work—and could I now fix it?

Mama cleared her throat. "There isn't much time until I start. We need to find care for Frits and Jean-Jean until they can go to *het kindertehuis.*"

Papa's eyes were glued to Jan as he answered. "They're good boys, and Marijke is still here. We can delay my first treatment, and I can do it. Please don't deprive me of these two months."

"Okay then. If you insist. I think it'll probably work because it's only for a short time. Of course, you won't be able to manage much longer than that."

A few days later, it was time to crystalize the plans. "So, how will we do this?" Papa fell back into his chair by the *kachel*, and I ran to snuggle on his lap. He absent-mindedly finger-combed my tangled curls.

"I explained our situation to our families," Mama replied. "My mother said she doesn't mind stopping in to see how you're doing. My brother, Henri, offered to drive you to your physician appointments and treatments, and his wife, Esther, said she'd help cook. Hearing about our predicament, even some neighbors offered to lend a hand if needed. And there's always your brothers and sisters. I hate to accept charity, but what choice do we have?"

I couldn't help interrupting. "Will Oom Henri and Tante Esther bring Meriam and baby Edith?" Our cousins were near in age to Jan and me, and despite being girls and not speaking French, they were good playmates.

Papa gently swatted my behind. "Toni, run off and let Mama and Papa talk. We'll figure out those very important details another time."

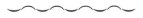

Waking up later than usual, I struggled into my layers of clothing and wandered into the kitchen. Mama had already left for work, and Papa was standing by the stove making coffee and our breakfast: bread, butter, and sugar, all soaked in warm milk. Jan was in his high chair, pretending the pieces of Edam cheese on his tray were cars.

With his warm smile lighting up his face, Papa patted my bottom. "Tuck your shirt in, Toni. Why's that so hard for you to remember? Then, sit down next to Jean-Jean. Breakfast is nearly ready."

"What are we going to do today, Papa?"

"Mama bought the food for tonight yesterday, so how about a walk in Westbroekpark? It's too cold for the beach."

Immediately, Jan began clapping his hands. Although he wasn't saying much yet, he clearly understood everything. Noticing that my hands were twirling, I quickly stuffed them in my pockets.

Papa chuckled. He never told me to *doe gewoon*. "I guess you're excited about that. And Jean-Jean certainly remembers chasing ducks from last week."

Caught up in the story, my arms and legs stiffened, and I began bouncing. "It was so funny. He chased them right into the lake! And then fell in himself." I turned to my brother. "Remember?"

Jan's eyes became saucers. "Coat wet. Shoes wet. Bad ducks!"

Papa threw back his head and guffawed. "I don't think it was the ducks' fault. Still, how about we don't do it again?"

With Jan in the stroller so that he wouldn't run to the lake, I danced beside Papa as he ambled through the meadows, flowers, and trees of the 44-acre Westbroekpark. Only when the wind had chapped our cheeks and turned our noses into cherries was it time to go home. Papa struggled up the stairs, leaving the stroller behind. After putting Jan down for a nap, he collapsed into his chair.

"Fritsje, please find Marijke and ask her to bring in the stroller. Then get Papa some bread and cheese. I'm hungry but just too tired to do it."

Lifting my chin, I told her about the stroller but not the lunch. I could do that myself. I dragged a chair over to the counter, got out a plate, and put butter on two slices of bread. Now to cut the cheese. With my tongue sticking out the side of my mouth, I pressed onto the Edam with a knife I'd found in the drawer.

"Fritsje!" Marijke shrieked. "Put down the knife! You know that's not allowed."

My lower lip trembled as my eyes filled. "I...I...I was making Papa *een boterham* (an open-faced sandwich)."

Her eyes crinkled in a way that reminded me of Mathieu. "I see. Let me help you with the cutting. You can do the rest." She quickly sliced the cheese and put it in a little pile on a plate in front of me.

I carefully placed Edam on top of the chunks of butter, smiling because Papa would be so impressed. After climbing down from my perch, I used both hands as I'd been taught and carried the plate with *boterhammen* to his chair. Marijke brought the cutlery. Papa was fast asleep.

Shrugging, I arranged the plate, knife, and fork on the table next to him. He'd see them when he awoke. Now, would he mind if I made myself some food? My tummy was rumbling. *Nee* (no), he never got mad about things like that. Unlike Mama. I made *een boterham* for myself, carefully swiping the crumbs onto the floor when I was done.

Mama hated it when the counters were dirty. I hoped that if I was helpful enough, she might decide to love me.

Rrriiinnng! I glanced around. Evidently, Marijke had gone upstairs, so it was up to me. After looking out the window to see if I recognized who was at the door, I ran to open it. "*Goedenavond, Mevrouw Beekhof,*" I said in my best Dutch before continuing in French. "I'm sorry, but Mama is at work, and Papa and Jan are asleep."

Mevrouw Beekhof looked a little confused. "Yes, of course."

I could see she didn't know what I'd said but still couldn't speak much Dutch, so I shrugged helplessly.

"Can you manage to take this basket of food up the stairs? I hoped it might help."

My nose was twitching with delight as I accepted the offering she held out to me. "*Oui,* I'm a big boy now. I can do it. Thank you!"

I soon grew used to our seemingly carefree routine. On warm mornings during the week, Papa took us to the beach. He and Jan built sand castles, and I waded in the icy water and watched crabs skitter into the sand.

If it was colder, we wore our coats and went to the Scheveningse bosjes. Jan picked up pine cones, sticks, stones, and various insects to show Papa, who strolled with his hands clasped behind him. Determined to impress my father with what a big boy I was, I copied him, putting my hands behind my back. I loved breathing deeply while listening to the crunch underfoot and watching how the sunlight played on the leaves. It's likely that, through this experience, I gained what would become much-needed knowledge: forests provide peace amidst turmoil.

The walk back home was always much slower; Papa was tired, an unwelcome reminder that he was actually very sick. Some days, his legs would give out, and I had to help him to bed. After lunch, I would look at books, do puzzles, tinker, and perhaps open the door to Tante Aleida or a kindly neighbor. Once she'd put Jan down, Marijke had her list of chores, and my time was my own.

My favorite visitors were Tante Esther and her girls. It was Tuesday, the day for her weekly visit, so I knelt by the window watching until I saw them coming.

With her dark hair and sparkling black eyes, my chubby-cheeked aunt huffed her way up our stairs carrying a pot of chicken soup with matzo balls. It smelled heavenly, and my mouth began to water.

Once it was safely simmering in the kitchen, Tante Esther bustled around plumping pillows and cleaning. She didn't notice

Meriam, Edith, Jan, and me giggling as we hid under the big table. At first.

"Shoo, *kindertjes* (little children). It's a lovely day. Go outside to play so you're not under my feet. Frits and Meriam, watch that Edith and Jan don't go too far."

We older children helped the younger ones into their coats, and we all ran down the stairs, me with a ball in hand. Cars were a rarity in those days, so playing in the street (there were no yards) was much safer than it might seem.

"Meriam, you have Jan on your team, and I'll have Edith on mine. That way, it'll be fair." I indicated what I meant with my hands since Meriam only spoke Dutch with the odd Yiddish word. By now, I understood most of what was said in Dutch but found it more difficult to speak.

Meriam put her hand on her hip. "Why?" That needed no interpretation.

I rolled my eyes and almost beat on my chest. "Obviously, because boys are better at ball games than girls." Truth be told, I wasn't very good at playing ball, having inherited a total inability to catch from my father's side of the family. But she didn't need to know that.

It was probably just as well that Meriam obeyed—and that she didn't understand me.

While chasing the ball, I saw Mama slowly trudging up the street. Holding Jan's hand, I went to meet her. Mama offered me her cool cheek before scooping Jan up. She had no choice, given that he was jumping up and down in front of her with his arms in the air.

Mama, who'd been trying to teach me Dutch, greeted my cousins and then addressed me slowly while clearly enunciating. "Ah, I see Tante Esther is here. Have you had a good day?"

"*Oui*, Edith and I won the game!"

"Frits, say it in Dutch."

I tried, then continued in French, "Mama, can Edith and Meriam stay for dinner? Can they? Tante Esther always makes a lot. So can they?"

Mama shook her head as she reached through the mail slot to pull on the chain that opened our door. "She won't want to stay, Frits. Her Sabbath begins tonight."

"Why not? I could let her have my chair. I like her, Mama. She's so fat that her hugs are just so cozy and warm! I heard Papa call her 'Dicky.' That means fat, right? Oom Henri could come, too. I think Papa called him 'Hans.' But what's his name, really? Why isn't he fat? Why?"

Mama flushed as Tante Esther appeared at the top of the stairs. She was putting her coat on. "*Goedemiddag* (Good Afternoon), Esther." She then bent down and scolded me in a fierce whisper. "Frits! It's not polite to comment on your aunt's shape. Now, I want to hear no more about it. They will never eat with us. Never."

I was going to ask more, but Mama already had her hand over my mouth.

Later that evening, while Marijke was putting Jan to bed, I couldn't stop wondering about what Mama said.

"Papa, why don't Oom Henri and Tante Esther eat at our house?" It was very convenient that whenever Papa was awake, he sat quietly in his special chair next to the *kachel*. That meant I could crawl onto his lap and ask as many questions as I liked.

"That's a good question, Frits. It's because they're *Joden* (Jewish people). For them, our food, dishes, and cutlery are dirty. Well, kind of. They call it 'unclean.'"

"But Papa, Tante Esther washed them herself! I saw her."

Papa chuckled. "So she did, and I'm very thankful. But Tante Dicky believes it would offend God if she ate here."

I put my head on one side. I had enough Jewish playmates to know a little about how things worked. "Umm, if Oom Henri is *Joods* (Jewish), then Mama is, too? He's her brother. Right?"

"Yes, but I'm not. And we don't keep kosher."

"So why does Mama eat with us?"

Now Papa laughed until the tears rolled down his cheeks. "Oh Toni, Toni, you're too logical for me. Mama doesn't believe that God exists, whether He's *Joods*, Christian, or something else; she's a Humanist. So, I guess she doesn't care if she offends Him."

"Papa, do you think God is real?"

Papa pursed his lips and shook his head. "I don't know. With all that's going on now, I doubt it. Probably not."

Since I had the security of my beloved Papa, a cozy home, and plenty of food, that conclusion didn't particularly bother me. Just after my fifth birthday, however, that was to change. Then, when memories were all I had to sustain me, I could have used a god. But my parents said God wasn't real. And they should know.

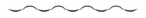

Sitting under the table trying to magnetize some metal, my attention was drawn by Mama whispering into the phone. "Mama, how do I do it? I just don't know how." A couple of minutes of listening. "*Ja* (yes), I know I need to tell him. I hate to, but I will. Okay, bye."

This sounded serious. When I heard her hang up, I crawled out and stood with my hands behind my back, watching her carefully. Mama had her head on the table. Was she sleeping, like Papa always did? No. Her shoulders were shaking. "Mama?"

After a few minutes, Mama lifted her head, seeming unaware of her wet cheeks. "Oh, there you are, Frits. Ask Mademoiselle Marijke to get Mama a drink, would you?"

I knew what she meant and watched Marijke quickly get her a glass of wine. That always seemed to make Mama feel better, at least for a little while. Recently, she'd needed a drink every day. I wasn't sure why since, when I'd secretly tried a drop left at the bottom of her glass, I found it tasted terrible.

The following weekend, just after Jan had been put to bed, I crawled under the table to quietly examine Papa's watch. How did it work? Why did the hands go around, and why did they stop if he forgot to wind it?

Mama came down the stairs and approached Papa, who was snoring in his chair, his head back and mouth open. She didn't see me since the tablecloth hid me from view.

"Freddie, wake up. We need to talk."

I held my breath. The stress of our lifestyle was taking a toll on my parents. They filled every weekend with shouted arguments. I was worried that Mama would once again begin with a litany of complaints. But she sounded despondent, not cross. She drew her chair up next to Papa and took his hand. I peeked out to see what was happening.

"What is it, *ma chéri*? You look so worried."

Mama's eyes darkened, and her shoulders grew round. "I didn't want to tell you, but my mother said I must. It's time."

"What?" Papa sometimes found it challenging to keep his eyes open all the way, making him look perpetually sleepy. However, his voice told me he was paying close attention. So was I.

"Dokter Smit called me into his office the other day. He told me more about your illness than he revealed originally. I didn't want to tell you because it's not good news…"

Papa smiled and covered her hand with his. "I know that I'll be lame despite the treatment. Don't worry…"

"Let me finish. This is hard enough!" Mama drew in a deep breath and continued. Her voice was shaky. "He said myasthenia gravis damages the muscles all over the body, not just the ones in eyes and legs. Eventually, it'll reach the muscles that help you breathe." She paused briefly before plowing on. "Well, I'm sure you can figure out what that means. He said it could take ten years, but it's much more likely to be fewer than four."

Papa squeezed his eyes shut. "I'm dying?"

Mama now looked like a deflated balloon. "*Oui, mon chéri.* You probably have four years."

It felt like a knife had pierced my chest, and I couldn't breathe. Although four years seems like a very long time when a person is only five, my world turned as gray as the weather. But not as black as it would.

She continued, "In October, Dokter Smit wants you to undergo some more treatments in the hospital in Leiden, followed by a spell in a rest home. But in the long run, I'm afraid it won't help. Nothing can save you."

Papa's voice came out as a squeak. "I see. I'm going to die. My time is running out."

"Probably," Mama whispered. "Although we can't lose hope."

Papa looked skyward before continuing with a wry smile. "I'm not sure what to hope for—a fast death or a slow and lingering one. Suffocation…"

Seeming not to hear him, Mama continued. "We need to prepare." She'd entered the organizer mode, which was far more familiar to me than the gentleness I'd just witnessed.

My heart was in my throat. How could this be? My loving and vital father would die? Pulling my knees up to my chest, I continued to listen carefully.

Papa passed his hands over his face. "Rita, this is an awful lot to take in. Can preparing wait until tomorrow? Maybe even next week? Please?"

"Fine. I'll go see Marijke about dinner." Mama turned on her heel, not even offering her trembling husband a hug.

I crawled out from under the table and climbed onto Papa's lap. We didn't need words as I wound my arms around his neck, and, with clouded eyes, he stroked my hair. In no time, he was again asleep. But I wasn't. How could it be that we could wind a watch but not a person? It sounded like there was nothing anyone could do.

A week later, I heard Mama and Papa talking in lowered voices. Could there be more bad news? It hardly seemed possible, and I was sure I didn't want to know. Nonetheless, I crept closer so I could hear.

"*Ma chéri*, you know I had to tell my employer that my illness is terminal? Well, I received his response today."

"What did he write?"

Papa blew up his cheeks and exhaled noisily. "He was very kind in the letter but said they have no choice. My job is over. I'll resign so they won't have to fire me. That means my sick pay will be terminated."

"Then, I guess it's a good thing I found that job. I just hope we'll be able to make ends meet."

Frits's and Jan's portrait done before leaving Aketi, 1937. (top)

Frits and Jan arrive in the Netherlands, January, 1938. (bottom)

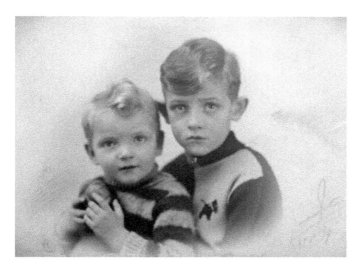

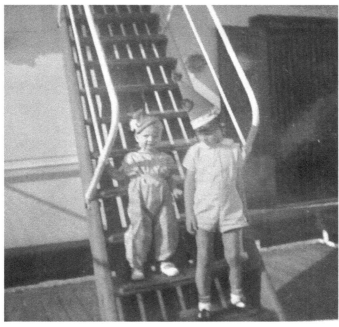

Papa and Frits go for a boat ride, August 1938. (top)

Tante Aleida and Frits at the seaside, July 1939. (bottom)

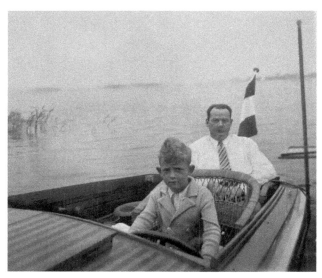

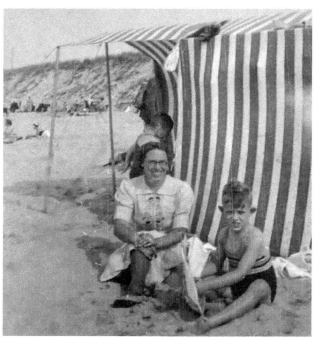

4

THE CHILDREN'S HOME

The squirrels were burying nuts, and the birds migrating south, signaling that our summer with Papa was over. The dreaded day was here. Since Papa was now in the hospital, it was Mama, Jan, and I who boarded the train to Driebergen. Our love-filled home overlooking the sea was to become only a memory.

I sat with my arms crossed over my stomach and my nose pressed to the window. Jan slept on the bench next to me, his head pillowed on his chubby arm. We passed lakes, canals, forests, and fields. Was this place on the other side of the world? It seemed like we'd been traveling for hours. How would I ever see Papa again? I swallowed hard, and a tear snaked its way down my cheek.

Finally, Mama put her book down, rose from her seat, and placed sleepy Jan on the floor. He wavered, and I jumped up and grabbed him lest he fall. "Okay, boys. We're here. Fritsje, you hold Jean-Jean's hand while I get the case."

It wasn't far to de Viersprong, Arnhemsebovenweg 40, which turned out to be a stately red-bricked mansion even bigger than our home in the Congo. I leaned back to count. It had three floors and seven windows just in the front! Maybe it would have boys…

Mama pulled the shiny bell, and the ornately carved wooden door creaked open. A nurse in a blue dress, starched white apron, and large stiff white cap stood there. She smelled of disinfectant. After looking down her long nose at each of us and checking the pocket watch attached to her apron, she intoned, "Ah, you must be Mevrouw Evenblij. Just in time. I'm Zuster Suus Dermout. It's nice to finally make your acquaintance in person. Come in, *alstublieft* (please)."

Zuster Dermout stepped back to allow us to enter the door that we soon learned was strictly forbidden to children. We all wiped our feet

41

in the vestibule before she led us through a wide corridor with an enormous staircase to the left. On the right, there was a doorway leading to the living room. With a slight motion of her bony hand, Zuster Dermout indicated we should precede her into that room. I looked around with interest at the elegant but old-fashioned furniture and the massive fireplace. An Axminster rug partly covered the highly polished wooden floor. Between us and the front window was a conservatory, which housed several house plants and even an orange tree. It was just as well that I filled my eyes then since that room and the conservatory were also totally off-limits to the younger inhabitants of the home.

"Have a seat, Mevrouw Evenblij."

Smoothing her skirt over her behind, Mama sat on the sofa, which was covered in itchy-looking brown fabric. The nurse then perched at the edge of a straight-backed chair, her legs pressed together and her ankles crossed. Jan and I remained standing.

On the way here, Mama said Jan and I would join about a dozen other children, but I'd neither seen nor heard anything that would betray their presence. I opened my mouth to ask Mama, but Zuster Dermout answered my unspoken question.

"The other *kinderen* (children) aren't here right now. My colleague, Zuster Mien Deenik, took them to *het bos* to pick beechnuts."

That would explain it. Maybe this place wouldn't be so bad. I gave Jan a cautious smile.

Zuster Dermout adjusted her wire-rimmed glasses and turned to observe Jan and me with the expression Mama sported when she saw an insect. "Introduce us, *alstublieft*. Who are these *kindertjes*?"

Mama drew Jan to her side. "This is Jan, but we call him Jean-Jean, and that's Fritsje."

I stood apart, chin thrust out and arms folded across my chest. I was brave and tough; nothing would hurt me!

"*Goedemiddag*, Jan and Frits." There was no warmth in Zuster Dermout's piercing voice. "Go sit over there on the floor while your mother and I talk. I'll show you the playroom and where you'll sleep forthwith."

I gazed silently at the tall sister, whose thin hair was tightly tucked into a bun at the back of her scraggly neck. Her mouth smiled, but not her slate-colored eyes. Even the roaring fire in the grate couldn't banish my goosebumps.

"Mevrouw Evenblij, I understand that you're working and living in Den Haag but seeking employment in Zeist."

"Yes, I want to be nearby."

Zuster Dermout continued as if Mama hadn't spoken. "Nevertheless, we find *kinderen* settle better if they do not see their parents for a month after coming to live with us. After that, you may only visit the boys for an hour on Sunday afternoons. I trust that's acceptable to you."

"*Ja*, Zuster Dermout, it's fine. I doubt I'll be able to visit more than twice a year, anyway. You will remember that I have an ailing husband."

"Of course," Zuster Dermout murmured.

Mama opened her purse. "Can I pay you for the first month now?"

Zuster Dermout's pinched nostrils flared slightly. "*Ja zeker* (yes, of course)." She continued in an oily tone of voice. "I understand you won't be able to pay us in full. We, of course, want to help in any way we can, so are most willing for Frits to work to make up the remainder of the cost of his and Jan's care."

"Of course. You're so kind and very generous. I'm grateful to leave the boys in your capable hands. What chores, specifically, will he be doing?" Mama examined her nails, ignoring me as I moved behind Zuster Dermout's back to pull faces at my little brother.

"Oh, we'll start easy. He'll just be polishing shoes on Saturdays and taking out some garbage. We'll add to his responsibilities as he gets older."

Mama nodded and narrowed her eyes at me in a silent warning. "Thank you for your understanding, Zuster Dermout."

Zuster Dermout gave a slight nod before she rose, giving off another whiff of disinfectant. "If you'll follow me to the other end of the hall, I'll show you the playroom and kitchen. There's a toilet there, but that's forbidden to *kinderen*."

A playroom? How wonderful! I quickly pulled Jean-Jean to his feet so I could follow closely. I held my breath as Zuster Dermout opened the door to reveal a spacious room with a large window facing the backyard on one side and a *kachel* on the other. Over the *kachel*, in pride of place, was the huge and ornate chiming clock that would henceforth rule my life.

On another side of the room was a wooden cabinet with shelves. Zuster Dermout told Mama that this is where each child can keep their special toys.

"Zuster Dermout, we didn't bring any toys," I said.

Zuster Dermout's stiff posture and refusal to look at me communicated that I'd done something wrong, but I wasn't sure what.

"Um, we can bring some next time we…," I started to add.

As if she hadn't heard, the haughty woman addressed Mama. "*Kinderen* who don't have toys here can play with those others have left behind. Provided, of course, that the parents give their permission."

I nodded in understanding, even though she still wasn't talking to me.

In the middle of the room was a massive wooden table. The nurse explained this was where children were to eat, do homework, and play. The ebony satin grand piano with its ivory keys was along the wall between the window and the door. While the two women spoke, I edged over to press on a key.

"*Kinderen* must have permission to touch the piano," Zuster Dermout barked.

I quickly put the offending hand behind my back.

Now that we'd been in that room for what Zuster Dermout deemed sufficient time, she closed the door and turned on her heel.

"Here's the kitchen. If you go through it, you'll see the cloakroom where *kinderen* hang their coats and the toilet they're allowed to use." Frowning, she bent to catch Jan's and my eye. "Be sure you never use the other one. Never."

Jean-Jean hid behind Mama, but I giggled. "That's okay. Jean-Jean usually goes in his pants, anyway."

Mama gasped. Zuster Dermout again acted as if she hadn't heard me. Strange. Maybe she couldn't understand French.

My eyes grew round as I caught sight of a monstrosity on the other side of the kitchen. "Jean-Jean," I whispered. "Just look at that huge black stove! It's as big as one of our rooms in Scheveningen!"

Zuster Dermout sniffed. "We only speak Dutch here, Frits. And *kinderen* should be seen and not heard."

So that was why she kept ignoring me! I made a mental note. Talking to the nurses was forbidden.

"Come with me up the stairs, Mevrouw Evenblij; I'll show you the bedrooms."

We walked back down the corridor toward the front door and ascended the wide staircase. At the top was another square hall with various doors. One led to the nurses' bedroom and another to a bathroom. Three doors opened into totally unheated bedrooms, each containing four bunk beds and two small chests of drawers. One room had pink curtains and was for the older girls; another had blue curtains and was for the older boys; and the final one had green curtains and was for the younger children.

"Frits and Jan will sleep in the green room."

I breathed a sigh of relief, having been worried that my little brother would have to sleep in a room without me.

Mama gazed up the next staircase. "What's up there?"

"Oh, just the laundry room, another bathroom, and a few smaller bedrooms. In case we take in more *kinderen*. Right now, we do not need it."

"Very good. Thank you for the tour, Zuster Dermout. I'd like to take a picture of the boys in the conservatory for my husband, and then I'll take my leave of you."

After regally descending the stairs and taking the photo, Mama shook the sister's hand. She then turned to us. "Frits, you may give me a kiss." She offered me her cool cheek, and I obeyed, hoping she'd rub my head like Papa would have. Instead, Mama patted Jan's curly head. "Be good, Jean-Jean."

And then she was gone. Jan silently put his finger in his mouth. As Mama closed the door, I remembered her words to Papa, and my breath came faster. Since she'd never wanted us, would she ever come back? I couldn't bear the idea of living here forever and grabbed the door handle to run after her.

Zuster Dermout pried my white fingers from the door and locked it. I backed up until I hit the wall, but she ignored the panic of the little boy in the foyer.

"Come, boys." She picked up our case and led the way back up the stairs to the green room, which I now noticed had no pictures on the walls. None!

"This bunk is where you'll sleep, Frits on the top and Jan on the bottom." I eyed the thin mattress, flat pillow, starched sheets, and brown woolen blankets, and a chill went down my spine. Cozy was not a word I would use.

"Frits, you can unpack Jan's and your *koffer* (suitcase) into this dresser. When you're finished, since you missed lunch, you can both come to the kitchen for some milk."

And so, she left me alone with my baby brother in a cold room in a strange house in a town far from my beloved Papa, knowing I would never see Mathieu and Yohan again. The earthquake of loss overwhelmed me, but even then, I knew I was the only one who could pull me out of the rubble.

"Frits," I told myself sternly, "do what Papa said. Be good and take care of Jean-Jean. And one day, you'll be allowed to go home."

Struggling with my small fingers, I opened what had once been Papa's *koffer*. Jan's clothing was neatly folded on one side and mine on the other. I remembered watching Marijke pack it and felt a wave of homesickness. Pulling open the drawers, I tried to remember how our clothes had been arranged at home. In the end, I opted for underclothes and socks in one drawer and outer garments in the other. I tried to keep the neat folds but, having never been taught, was sure Zuster Dermout would be dissatisfied with my efforts. Last, I tucked the magnet and the crystal I'd smuggled from home under my clothing.

The sound of childish voices began floating up the stairs. Strangely, I was sure I could also hear moans. Maybe better not to go down yet! I slid to sit on the floor beside our bunk. Being engrossed in figuring out how the latch of the *koffer* worked, Jan didn't seem to notice the noises.

Just then, the door opened, seemingly of its own accord. In walked a small brown and white dog with outlandishly long ears. "Come here, boy," I whispered, causing Jan to look up and gasp. "Don't worry. He's a friendly dog, Jean-Jean. Look!" I pulled the mutt onto my lap and buried my face in his fur. Jan curled up beside us. That's how we sat for the rest of the afternoon.

"Frits and Jan, come down now. It's dinner time." Zuster Dermout's voice became even more harsh when it was raised.

I crept down the wooden stairs, clutching my brother's hand, to be greeted by a rather rotund sister, also dressed in blue and white and smelling of disinfectant. Her pale blue eyes crinkled a welcome, but I was in no mood for pleasantries.

"Hello. You must be Frits. I'm Zuster Deenik. Come with me. In the future, you must remember that dinner is at 6:00 pm."

My eyes grew as big as saucers when we reached the playroom. The room was full of children, but they were silent.

At two years old, Jan was the youngest of the children by far. Most of them looked like they were between 8 and 12 years old. "I'll sit here, Jean-Jean," I whispered as I took the seat next to my little brother 's high chair.

"Mama? Papa? When come?"

I shook my head sadly. "They're not coming, but don't worry. Fritsje will take care of you."

"Silence!" Zuster Dermout shot daggers out of her eyes. It seemed that conversing in French would not be a problem; even speaking to other children was prohibited.

Fortunately, Jan was quickly distracted by the boiled potatoes, Belgian endive, chicken, and milk placed in front of him. I noticed that female staff, not houseboys, brought out the food, shattering my only hope of receiving some love in this place.

My eyes were attracted to a boy at the other end of the table, who was repeating "silence" over and over again while flapping his arms.

"That's Jantje. There's something very wrong with him, but he's the sisters' favorite. He even sleeps in their room," Appie, the boy who was sitting next to me, whispered. "Don't look at him."

I put my head down and silently ate my food.

"Frits! Sit up straight. Bring your food to your mouth, not your mouth to the food."

I cocked my head to one side, mulling this over. Surely, both actions would result in the same thing—the food would go in your mouth. But the sister's lips were pressed together. Apparently, even when I wasn't trying to offend, in this place, I would. Glancing at the child across from me, I imitated his posture and managed to get through until the meal ended. 6:30 pm.

"Upstairs; clothes off." What could Zuster Deenik mean? Astonished, I opened my mouth to ask, but an older boy, Hans, shook his head at me. Of course. We weren't allowed to speak to the sisters unless first spoken to. So, I watched.

Standing on the upstairs landing outside the unheated bathroom, all the children ten years old and under removed their clothing. I could do that. After taking mine off, I helped Jean-Jean and looked around to see what would happen next.

The children stood in a line, naked, goosebumps plainly in evidence. Then, one at a time, we were ushered into a bathtub filled with rather cloudy, lukewarm water. Since everyone else seemed to accept this, I submitted to being washed by Zuster Dermout and dried by Zuster Deenik. Their scaly hands on my body reminded me of how soft and gentle my father's hands always felt. But Papa wasn't there, and this was to happen every night without fail.

That evening, after helping Jan into his pajamas and tucking him in, I climbed onto the top bunk. The sound of snuffling and movement from the other children was magnified in the darkness, and I felt panic building in my chest. How would I survive this? How could I take care of Jean-Jean here? Would I ever see Papa again? The pounding of my heart echoed in my ears, and I started to gasp for breath. My feet crept toward the side of the bed as I prepared to escape…

"Hey, Frits! That's your name, right?"

I turned toward the whisperer in the next bunk.

47

"Yeah. Who are you?"

"I'm Dirk. I'm nearly six, and my mom says I'm trouble."

I was not alone. I grinned into the darkness while speaking my best Dutch. "Pleased to meet you, Trouble."

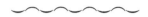

The discordant ringing of a bell rudely threw me from where I'd been riding on Yohan's shoulders under a sunny, cerulean sky into a hard bed in a cold and shadowy room. It was 6:00 am.

Dirk hopped down from the top bunk next to me and showed me what I had to do for Jan and myself. I washed our faces with the cold water in the communal bowl and combed our curls. After I was dressed in my gray shorts, shirt, knee socks, and woolen sweater, I helped Jan into his.

Dirk wriggled his eyebrows at me. "Now, we go downstairs to the toilet to do a big one."

"Do you mean…?"

"Yup!" Dirk's grin split his face.

"What? On command? What if I don't have to go?"

"Do it anyway. It makes them happy. If you do it later, they'll beat you with the *mattenklopper* (carpet beater)." Dirk shoved me playfully.

"Really?"

His smile faded. "*Jawel* (yes, of course*).*"

So, holding Jan's hand, I followed Dirk and the others down to take turns in the bathroom. I turned red and was finally successful, but Jan wasn't. I hoped they'd be merciful to the little guy.

Finally, it was 7:30 am. Breakfast time. After a prayer, the kitchen staff gave us buttered bread, boiled eggs, and milk. I watched and copied the bigger children, who all took their fork in their left hand and their knife in their right to cut their bread into four strips. They cut each strip into six pieces. Finally, each piece was speared with their fork and carefully and thoroughly chewed before they took another bite.

The nurses focused eagle eyes on us to be sure no one deviated from the mandated procedure. It was weird but not so terrible. Boiled eggs were my favorite, and at least we didn't have to cut those into strips!

No sooner had we said the after-breakfast prayer than Zuster Dermout beckoned me toward her. I glanced anxiously at Jan. Should I

48

bring him? After all, Papa always told me it was my responsibility to take care of him. Not to do so would be unforgivable, wouldn't it?

"Never mind your *broertje* (little brother), Frits. Your job is to earn his and your keep through hard work. No complaining. No shirking. And no half-jobs. I'll only show you once, so pay attention."

As she spoke, Zuster Dermout strode ahead of me, out the back door, through the small garden, and around to the side of the building. She stopped just behind the bicycle shed and garage. Although this position provided some shelter from the wind, rain drizzled down my neck, making me shiver. The sister seemed impervious to the weather, standing straight and stiff as she spat out her orders. Maybe she was made of stone?

"This is the garbage can. Every day after breakfast, you will empty the garbage from the upstairs hall, the playroom, and the kitchen. Empty it into here."

I was motionless as questions zoomed around in my head. I already knew that asking them was forbidden, so just hoped I'd somehow figure out the answers.

"Well, don't just stand there! Do it. Now! While I'm watching. After that, you're on your own, but I won't tolerate any incomplete work."

As the sister continued speaking in her abrasive voice, my eyes grew wider before my legs began moving. The very thought of touching garbage made me sick to my stomach. I wondered if she would allow me to wash my hands three times afterward like I always did at home. If not, I'd have to figure out a way to do it while she wasn't looking.

"Now! What are you waiting for?"

"Um, Zuster Dermout, which do I do first?" I hoped that I was permitted to answer since she asked me a question.

The ill-tempered woman snorted before she led the way. The cans from the playroom and hall weren't too bad, but the kitchen trash was both smelly and heavy. Tipping it slightly, I dragged it out the door and to the outside receptacles. But how could I get the garbage from one can to the other? I glanced up at Zuster Dermout, but her face had turned into granite. I was on my own.

Trying not to gag, I did what I had to do. Two handfuls at a time, I moved the foul contents of the kitchen trash can into the outdoor one until there was little enough left that I could lift the can. Then, holding my hands out from my sides, I went into the house and washed them at the cloakroom sink. Three times. Luckily, by then, Zuster Dermout had lost interest in tormenting her new mouse.

Poor little Jean-Jean was very unhappy all that first day. The sisters didn't allow me to stay by his side and totally ignored his tears. The sound of sobs and sniffles followed me wherever I went, and I felt my eyes welling up in sympathy. Hopefully, dinnertime would give him a break from their baptism by fire.

That night, I learned my next lesson: a person must always finish their meal, regardless of whether they like what's served. We were having cabbage for dinner, something Jean-Jean particularly hated. Pushing his little body as close to me as he dared, Jan ate everything on his plate except the disgustingly overcooked vegetable.

I noticed Zuster Dermout watching us, but she said nothing. Maybe she would have mercy? No. Instead, she motioned to the kitchen lady, and when it was time for dessert (porridge), the lady poured the sticky mess over Jan's cabbage.

Zuster Dermout then drew near and issued her instruction, emphasizing each word with stiffened lips. "Eat. Every. Bite." She didn't need to say, "or else."

Her pale eyes lit up with malicious pleasure as she watched my little brother struggle, gagging. Fortunately, she occasionally looked away, allowing me to reach over and take surreptitious bites of the revolting mixture. Finally, it was gone. Papa would've been proud.

On Saturday, Zuster Dermout showed me my next job. Once a week, before dinner, all the children at *het kindertehuis* lined their shoes up in the cloakroom by the back door. I added ours to the line and was just going to pick a whimpering Jan up when I heard, "Frits, leave him. The sooner he gets used to being alone, the better. You follow me."

"Zuster Dermout, I'll come as soon as he's settled."

"*Nee*, you'll come now. Shoes must be cleaned at 5:00 pm precisely. And you're going to do it."

"But Papa told me I have to take care of him. This is only his sixth day ever away from home!" Tears of panic sprung to my eyes; this was my duty, and it was important.

At this, the woman blew up to look even more menacing than she already was, and her piercing voice stabbed holes in my heart. "What? You dare to talk back to me? And even argue?"

I fell onto my bottom from the force of her slap across my face. The pain overflowed onto my cheeks. The sisters were, after all, our caretakers, and I hoped I could somehow earn their love.

"Get up, you clumsy child. Follow me."

From across the room, I heard Jean-Jean's voice. "No hit! Bad!"

Zuster Deenik scooped my brother up and took him away, even as he continued screaming and pounding his little fists on her back.

"Leave him alone!" I shouted before scrambling to my feet.

Zuster Dermout's fingernails dug into my arm as she, too, manhandled an Evenblij boy. Once we reached the back hall, she showed me the shoe-cleaning tools. "Do you know how to polish shoes, *jongeman*?"

Massaging my bruised arm, I scrunched up my nose and shook my head sulkily. "The houseboys or Papa did that at home."

"Stupid spoiled child! I'll show you once. After that, you'll do it and do it well. Every week without fail."

"*Ja*, Zuster Dermout. *Bedankt*." I hoped the sisters might be kinder to my little brother and me if I was outwardly submissive.

After demonstrating on one pair of shoes, Zuster Dermout went to sit with the older children in the playroom. I crouched on the drafty floor, polishing, and polishing, before carefully lining the shoes up from biggest to smallest. Then I went to wash my hands. Three times.

The initial weeks at *het kindertehuis* continued in the same vein as we gradually learned what was expected and what wasn't allowed. Poor Jan often cried himself to sleep, just wanting a goodnight embrace. I wasn't permitted to do it since the sisters forbade getting out of bed, even if a person needed the bathroom.

Fortunately, if Jan's weeping became too loud, Trouble would tiptoe to the door and keep watch. I would then creep down from my bunk to give my brother a quick hug, which I said came from Papa.

Don't get me wrong. I did get used to it. And while very strict, the routine of *het kindertehuis* wasn't all bad. As Mama had promised, we often went on excursions. When it was warm, and nothing else was planned, we went swimming. When it was cold, the sisters loaded the smaller children into a cart fastened to a bar under the saddle of Zuster Deenik's bike and to the harness of a large black sheepdog. In this fashion, the smaller children were pulled to some outing or other. The older ones got to ride their bikes, which looked like great fun to me.

"Hey, Frits, sit here over the wheel. That's where you get the best bumps!"

I laughed. "Maybe I don't want a red bottom like yours, Trouble. Where I was born, only the monkeys had red butts."

"Yeah, well, where I was born, only poodles have curly hair."

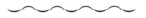

It was Sunday at 2:00 pm.

"Frits and Jan, once you've stacked your lunch plate on the side, wash your hands and face and go into the living room. Your mother is here to see you."

"Mama!" Jan's little legs were a blur as he ran down the hall toward our mother. I followed slowly. He had yet to learn that she wasn't a source of love.

Mama brushed a perfunctory kiss across Jan's cheek, and he climbed onto her lap.

"*Nee,* Jean-Jean. You'll wrinkle my skirt. Sit here on the floor at my feet." Mama then turned to me, who was standing in the doorway with my hands behind my back. "Hello Frits. It's nice to see you both. Have you been good boys?"

"Jean-Jean is, and I am…mostly." I shuffled my feet, knowing my honesty might get me into trouble.

Mama raised her shapely eyebrows.

"Sometimes I disobey the rules, and the sisters get mad at me." I pulled the door shut in case they were listening. "They hit me with the *mattenklopper;* it makes Jean-Jean cry."

Mama's lips pressed together before she heaved a sigh. "Well, Frits, if they're angry, I'm sure they have a good reason. You'll have to try harder."

"*Ja,* Mama. I will." I knew a façade of compliance was essential if this visit was to continue, and I was to receive an answer to my burning question. "How's Papa? Can we see him?"

"He's still in the hospital getting the medications he needs, but he'll soon be transferred to a rest home where he can recover. I brought you a letter from him. Can you read yet?"

"I'm still learning, Mama. Joined-up writing is hard. Can you read it to us, *alstublieft*?"

Mama nodded and unfolded the document. I sat at her feet with my chin in my hands. I listened to Papa's words, just imagining I was on his lap. How I missed him!

"Can I have it, Mama?" I asked once she'd finished reading.

She handed me the letter wordlessly. Taking it from her, I held it to my nose. Just as I'd suspected, it emitted Papa's fragrance. This would go in my secret box of special things.

"Well, I need to go if I'm to catch the next train. This has been lovely." Mama stood and began to put on her coat and gloves.

"Mama, take me! Don't go. *Alstublieft!*" Jan melted into a flood of tears and clung desperately to her leg.

"Frits, take your *broertje*."

After peeling his fingers off Mama, I held Jan's hand, knowing that crying wouldn't help. It only took a few more months for him to learn. Soon after Jan turned three, I never saw him cry again.

Mama visited us every three-to-six months during our first couple of years at *het kindertehuis*. Unless I knew Papa was coming with her, I did not look forward to the visits. Eventually, neither did Jan.

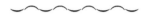

Visits that I did enjoy were those of Juffrouw (Miss) Meta van Kempen, the woman who would be my teacher. This wonderful lady sometimes came and taught the younger children while Jan napped. She quickly learned of my interest in magnets and light and often brought me some curiosity to examine.

One day, Juf van Kempen entered the playroom with an unnaturally pale face and rounded shoulders. She slumped into a chair by the table and put her head in her hands. Her long blond hair hid her face from her anxious observers, but we silently drew near.

I exchanged a glance with Trouble. Juf van Kempen was usually so engaged: guiding our little hands to form letters on a page, teaching us songs, and reading us stories. What was going on?

My courageous friend bent over to peek under her hair. "Why are you sad?"

Juf van Kempen looked up, and I was shocked to see her sky-blue eyes filled with rain. "I just heard something on the radio that's very upsetting. Bad, bad things are happening in Germany and Austria."

I looked at the map on the playroom wall. Our teacher had previously explained that Germany was the big gray country right next to our tiny orange one. Austria, which was blue, and Sudetenland, which was green, were on the other side of Germany. My mind began to wander. The Netherlands wasn't really orange. It was mostly gray in Den Haag and mostly green in Driebergen. So why did the map say it was orange?

"What happened?" asked Trouble, drawing my attention back to the conversation at hand.

Juf van Kempen shook her head. "I'm not sure if I should tell you, but I'm afraid you'll find out anyway." She sighed and whispered to herself, "Better they hear it from me," before continuing louder. "The radio said some angry men went out at night and broke windows in places where *Joden* live and work."

A blond urchin sitting across the table from me and beside my teacher raised her hand. "Breaking windows is bad, Juffrouw."

Juf van Kempen's face creased into a smile, and she stroked the girl's hair. "You're right. Breaking windows or breaking anything is wrong. She sighed. "But sometimes grown-ups do bad things."

I thought about how Zuster Dermout occasionally became frustrated enough to push me around. Once, I fell into a window. Granted, it didn't break, but it could have. So, I knew Juf van Kempen was right; even adults can break windows.

"Juffrouw, why did the men do that?" I asked. Could it be the Jews had been bad, just like Zuster Dermout so often said I was?

My teacher cast a quick glance around the playroom. "Remember that I told you a man called Adolf Hitler is in charge of Germany? Well, he said *Joden* caused all the bad things that are happening there. It's not true, but some people, called Nazis, believe Hitler's lies. Nazis really hate *Joden*."

"Teacher, lying is bad!" exclaimed the little girl.

"So is hating," offered Trouble.

My brow furrowed as I thought through what my teacher had said. This was worrying. I got up and crept close enough to lay a grubby hand on her knee. "*Joden* live in Driebergen, too. Do Nazis? Will the bad men break our windows?"

Juf van Kempen made the sign of the cross over her chest but didn't offer the reassurance her young and now frightened audience craved. "I don't know. Grown-up problems are complicated. Anyway, we don't need to talk more about it here. Do you have any books you'd like me to read?"

Later that afternoon, I crept into my hiding place behind the playroom curtain. I needed to think. Oom Henri, Tante Esther, and my cousins were Jews. Would the Nazis break the windows of the boarding house they ran? And what about Mama? Would they break her windows, too? Germany was right next to the Netherlands. Would the Nazis come here, or even worse, were they here already? I swallowed hard, trying to push down the butterflies that had taken up residence in my stomach.

"Frits! I see you there. Stop dawdling! It's time to get the potatoes from the cellar for dinner. Hurry, or I'll make you hurry." Zuster Deenik's gravelly voice told me that thinking time was over.

1939   It was just after dinner on Saturday, and a hush fell over the playroom because Zuster Deenik was holding a bunch of envelopes in her hands. Every child held their breath, hoping for news from family. It was all we had to comfort our lonely hearts, and we craved those letters more than the sweetest candy. My sixth birthday, the first in Driebergen, had been and gone with little notice. The sisters led a round of *Lang Zal Hij Leven* (a Dutch Happy Birthday song), but there was no cake. No visits. No gifts.

I listened carefully, my heart in my throat, as she called out name after name. Then, "Frits!" Zuster Deenik was holding a letter for me!

I jumped from my chair and ran.

"No running!"

Screeching to a sedate walk, I glanced up. Surely, that wasn't a smile playing around the edges of her mouth!

"Here you are. It looks like it's from your father."

Clutching the precious missive in my hand, I crept to sit behind the playroom curtain. Perhaps I could read the whole thing before being reminded to do one of my chores.

Lieve grote jongen van Papa en Mama (Sweet big boy belonging to Dad and Mom). Seeing those words on the page, my eyes welled with tears of relief. Papa always had so much love in his voice. Reading his words filled me up.

Drying my eyes, I continued.

> So, your birthday is finally here. It took so long—you were looking forward to it so much last time, my little boss. It's a shame Papa isn't better yet because then I would have quickly taken the diesel train so I could come to you today. Instead, you are getting a long letter from Papa, one that is only for you. That is also wonderful, isn't it, my sweet big boy?
>
> Yes, now you are six, you are starting to belong to the group of the bigger kids. Do you enjoy that? Or would you still like to be as small as your little brother? No, sweet Toni, now you are big, you'll soon be allowed to go to school. You will love that!
>
> Now, but first, Papa wants to wish his sweet Fritsje a happy birthday. Papa hopes you will be very good this year, also to Jean-Jean, even though he's sometimes mean to you. Remember, your little brother

is still a baby. Will you also continue to love Papa and Mama both the same, even though you don't see them very often now? We think about our eldest boy a lot, don't you know, my sweet little boss?

You must write and tell us if you had a lovely birthday. Ask Zuster Deenik or Zuster Dermout to help you write the letter. Did you have nice presents and maybe a tasty pastry? Maybe more than one? You would like that, you sweet candy-eater! But I know you didn't ask for a cake, since that's not allowed. No, of course not. Little children are not allowed to ask, but once you're six, you're absolutely not allowed to ask.

Mom said that Thea is also in Driebergen, and you must like that. Hey, Toni, say hi to her from Papa, and a kiss is also allowed, sweetheart. Whose sweetheart are you? Papa's and Mama's! You know that, don't you? Okay, sweet boy, if Zuster Dermout knows about a house for Papa in Driebergen, I'll come and live nearby for a while. Then maybe I'll see you soon again.

If I were with you now, I'd give you a big kiss with both your arms around Papa's neck. Give your sweet little brother also an extra hug, and, because it's your birthday, from Papa and Mama, also a lot of kisses.

Goodbye, my dear sweetheart,
from Papa and Mama

I carefully folded the letter and slipped it into my pocket before going to take the trash out. I remembered that Jean-Jean pulled my hair during Mama's last visit—and I'd reacted by pushing him so hard that he'd fallen over. That must be what Papa was referring to. Knowing that Mama told my father about my misbehavior, I resolved to do better in the future.

What about his request that I love both my parents equally? That was more difficult. How could I? Papa was the one who hugged and kissed me, the one who wrote to me, the one who called me a dear, sweet boy. Mama wasn't mean to me, but she sure wasn't warm. It would be nice if she loved her boys, but I was pretty certain she didn't. I shook my head. As much as I might want to, I could not and would not fake my feelings. Papa was my favorite. Always was. Always would be.

"Frits, now that you're six, you're old enough to take on another chore. Collecting firewood." Zuster Dermout's hard smile told me she thought I'd be upset. I was not.

I was to drag a wagon to the nearby forest and collect sticks and logs to feed the kitchen stove and the fireplace in the living room. Since the weather was often frosty, I got to do this chore almost every day.

I relished it! Being alone, listening to the wind rustle through the treetops, inhaling the fresh air, and examining white-spotted toadstools. If I had extra time, I even searched for orange-bellied newts to take back to Jan. The forest played a large part in keeping me sane as all control of my life was wrested out of my hands. Later, when the self-same chore became a source of great anxiety, the nurses deemed Jan old enough to help, so at least I had company.

Over the following months, tensions rose in Europe, and *het kindertehuis* began to fill up. One of the first children to come was the very talented Keet van Zanten. At only eight years old, Keetie was already an accomplished pianist. In the evening, after dinner, the sisters gave her permission to play the piano while the rest of us read, played games, or, in my case, did the chores to which I'd been assigned. The sweet notes both drowned out Jantje's strange screams and made my work pleasant as I lost myself in the music. Once I completed my tasks and washed my hands three times, I crept into the playroom and sat on the floor behind the piano bench, hoping Keetie wouldn't notice.

She did. At the end of a beautiful Viennese waltz, Keetie turned toward where I was sitting and addressed me in a voice that was almost as melodic as her playing. "Hey you, what's your name?"

Looking down, I mumbled, "Frits." Several children in the home had observed that I was the errand boy and scapegoat; they joined in with what they saw modeled by the sisters. I expected no different from Keetie.

"Well, Frits, come sit here." With her shiny black curls bouncing, Keetie grinned and patted the place beside her.

I could hardly believe my ears, but she didn't need to ask twice. I immediately climbed up, my bare legs swinging from the seat.

"Can I sit up there, too?" asked Trouble, raising a leg in anticipation.

Keetie winked at me. "Nope. Only Fritsje."

I took my place next to her, holding my breath during the fast pieces and covertly wiping my eyes throughout the slow. The music filled me until I overflowed. And the kind girl with her warm brown eyes understood.

The next day, I worked up the courage to ask Keetie something I'd been pondering during my chores. "D...d...do you think you could teach me to play?"

"I expect so. But we'll have to ask the sisters if it's allowed. And you'd have to practice."

I nodded furiously. "Oh, I will!"

"Then, I'll ask." Keetie bounced up to Zuster Dermout. "Would it be alright if I taught Fritsje how to play the piano?"

Zuster Dermout shook her head and pruned her lips. "You can try, but I have to tell you he's sometimes a very bad boy. I'm not sure he'll be an obedient pupil. He's difficult."

My shoulders slumped, but Keetie was undeterred. "Oh, that's okay. I always wanted a younger brother. Let me try. *Alstublieft?*"

"Of course. Just be sure that he doesn't neglect his duties."

"Yes, Zuster Dermout. I will." After turning away from Zuster Dermout, Keetie winked at me. I stifled my answering grin, but my heart grew warm.

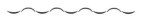

"Underpants check tonight!" Zuster Deenik narrowed her eyes while peering at the new children.

Keetie's eyes met mine, horror turning them into saucers. I knew what she was asking and whispered the answer.

"Umm, They do that sometimes. While waiting in line for our bath, we all have to hold our underpants in front of us so she can look inside."

"That sounds horrible. Why?"

I shrugged. "It's not so bad. She's checking for skid marks. If your pants are clean, it's fine. I'm sure yours are. It's only a problem if they're dirty. That's a big problem."

"How embarrassing! Does everyone have to do it?"

"Yup. Everyone except kids who wear diapers. And we don't have any of those now."

I frowned, noticing that Keetie was blinking back tears at the very thought of the upcoming humiliation. How could I help? I couldn't get her out of it. Perhaps I could distract her instead.

When the time came to get in line, I carefully positioned myself a few children down from Keetie. That way, Zuster Deenik's back faced me while Keetie's undies were checked. I was pretty proud of myself for this brilliant idea: I pulled faces at Keetie while it was happening. It was working well, judging by her sparkling eyes. At least, until Eddie pointed my antics out to Zuster Dermout.

"Frits! How can you be so disrespectful?" Zuster Dermout grabbed my arm before slapping me across the face, causing my nose to bleed.

"I...I...I..." I couldn't tell her why I'd done what I did.

Another slap followed, this time to my bare bottom. "Don't talk back!"

Jan, who was just behind me, watched in silent dismay.

"*Alstublieft*, zuster," I begged. "Let *mijn* (my) *broertje* go ahead. He's so little. And he's cold."

Zuster Dermout's face turned purple, and she hit me so hard that I fell against the wall. The young spectators were shocked into silence. I lay stunned for a few minutes before becoming aware of her piercing voice. "Get up. Clean up that blood! And learn your lesson."

Steam came out of my ears and my face flushed before I jumped up and shouted, "Oh, I've learned. I've learned that you're unfair and nasty!"

Of course, that earned me another blow, but at least I'd had my say and regained some of my dignity. As much as is possible when a person is naked. Now, with blood, tears, and snot dripping from my face, I submitted to being bathed and then slipped into my pajamas.

Once dressed, I limped to the kitchen to fetch a sponge to wash the wall. When I could finally go to Jan, he was naked and shaking under his covers.

"Jean-Jean, don't worry. I'm okay. She's just a stupid old witch."

"I'm c...c...cold. Zuster Dermout made me stand on the t...t...tile floor in my b...b...bare feet for a long time!"

"What? Why? That old meanie! I've seen her do that to other kids but never thought she'd do it to you! I'll show her!" My nostrils flared as my fists clenched.

Jan reached up to touch my face and whispered. "*Nee,* don't. *Alsjeblieft,* be good. I hate it when you hurt."

I gently rubbed his back. "*Bedankt*, little guy. Now, let's get you into your pajamas, and I'll hold you until you're warm again. Well, at least until we hear the witch coming in."

Once everyone was in bed and the lights were out, I heard a whisper from the bunk next to ours. "Frits, I don't know what all you did to make the old *gemenerik* (meanie) so mad, but don't do it again! That was scary. I thought she was going to kill you for sure!"

"*Bedankt*, Trouble. I'll keep your feelings in mind during future fights." I fell asleep with a grin on my very painful face.

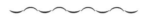

As happened every Sunday morning, a bell clanged through the hallways before it was even light. We'd all put our everyday clothes ready to be washed the previous night, so we dressed in our clean Sunday clothes and the shoes I'd shined. After the mandatory toilet session and breakfast, Zuster Dermout marched the older children to the *Grote Kerk* (big church) at the other end of Driebergen's main street, the Traaij. The younger ones, like Jan, got a ride in the cart. Jan was still afraid of dogs, but at least this one was busy pulling.

Distracted by the clocks in a shop front that we were passing, I didn't notice Keetie slow her march until she was walking beside me.

"Fritsje, Zuster Dermout said we're going to *de kerk*." She spoke under her breath since we weren't allowed to talk here either.

"Yeah, we are. Why?"

"Um, I'm *Joods*. I don't go to church. My parents sometimes took us to synagogue, but never church."

I stopped to think about this.

"Keep walking, Frits," she whispered. "They're looking."

"Okay," I answered slowly. "Well, I think that going to *de kerk* is a rule for living at *het kindertehuis*. My parents never went to church. But here, everyone goes, even if they're *Joods*, just like everybody has to say grace. If you don't like it, just don't listen to the pastor. I pretty much never do."

Keetie snickered, drawing the attention of the disciplinarian at the back of our line. "You're so funny. You remind me of my big brothers, Aron and Benjamin. Except you're much younger."

My chest puffed up at the idea that I reminded anyone of someone older than Keetie, and I swaggered a bit before whispering, "I'm glad we're friends."

"Me, too."

"Silence in the line!" Zuster Dermout was indeed watching.

Keetie took my hand before we continued down the street, entered the church, and slid into a pew at the back.

Just then, the organ started, the choir began singing, and my mouth dropped open. I reveled in the sound before I noticed the words. But then, they imprinted themselves on my heart.

Wat de toekomst brengen moge,
mij geleidt des Heren hand;
moedig sla ik dus de ogen
naar het onbekende land.

Leer mij volgen zonder vragen;
Vader, wat Gij doet is goed!
Leer mij slechts het heden dragen
met een rustig, kalme moed!

Heer, ik wil uw liefde loven,
al begrijpt mijn ziel U niet.
Zalig hij, die durft geloven,
ook wanneer het oog niet ziet.

Schijnen mij uw wegen duister,
zie, ik vraag U niet: waarom?
Eenmaal zie ik al uw luister
als ik in de hemel kom!

Laat mij niet mijn lot beslissen:
zo ik mocht, ik durfde niet.
Ach, hoe zou ik mij vergissen,
als Gij mij de keuze liet!

Whatever the future may bring,
The Lord's hand is leading me;
To the place that he's preparing,
I look to eternity.

Teach me, Father, now to trust you,
All your ways are good and right;
Help me know that all I must do,
Is to lean on Jesus Christ.

Lord, I praise your loving kindness,
Even when the darkness looms;
When my darkness turns to blindness,
I believe your light breaks through.

In my times of doubt and questions,
When I do not understand;
I rest in the hope of Heaven,
Where your glory fills the land!

In your hands I won't be shaken,
I submit my will to yours;
Oh, how I would be mistaken,
Not to trust you all the more.

Wil mij als een kind behand'len,
dat alleen de weg niet vindt:
neem mijn hand in uwe handen
en geleid mij als een kind.

Father, lead me as your child who,
Cannot find the way alone;
Take me in your arms, and I
Will follow till you call me home.

Waar de weg mij brengen moge,
aan des Vaders trouwe hand,
loop ik met gesloten ogen
naar het onbekende land.

Whatever the future may bring,
The Lord's hand is leading me;
I believe the Savior's promise,
Life with him eternally.

Turning to Keetie, I whispered, "What do you think the song means? Is there really a god who cares about us? Who we can trust?"

She shrugged. "Papa and Mama say there is. I guess they know. But it's not Jesus."

Now, it was my turn to shrug.

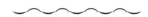

"Frits, Jan, come. Your parents are here to see you."

What? Papa was here? It'd been more than a year since we'd seen him, ever since we left home. Zuster Deenik hadn't succeeded in finding him a place nearby. Mama told us he'd been in hospitals and rest homes ever since we'd come to *het kindertehuis*. Entirely forgetting Jan, I ran to the living room, stopping short at the door.

Mama was seated on the couch, but who was this emaciated man in the wheelchair?

"Papa?" I queried, my voice trembling.

The man's face lit up with Papa's unique and wonderful smile, and he held out his arms. "Toni! It's so good to see you. Oh, and my Jean-Jean is here, too. What a wonderful, wonderful day for Papa!"

I quickly took my place by his side, inhaling his unique scent and enjoying the familiar feeling of him stroking my hair. Soon, I bubbled over with all the news that the sisters and Mama weren't interested in hearing.

"Papa, did you know I get to pick up sticks in *het bos* all by myself? That's because I'm a big boy. Also, I'm learning to play the piano. Keetie says I'm very talented. Am I?"

"*Ja*, you are, and I'm so proud of you. And what about Jean-Jean? Is he happy? Are you taking good care of him?"

I frowned and shuffled my feet. "Papa, I try, but sometimes I can't. Like when I'm doing the chores or the sisters lock me in the attic for punishment. It's really dark and scary there!"

A cloud passed over Papa's face. "Oh dear. I didn't know they do that—that's terrible. *Alsjeblieft*, do your very best to be good, my Toni, so that it won't happen again. About your *broertje*, I'm sure you're doing a great job."

Papa held his arms out to Jan. "Now, Jean-Jean, tell your papa. How are you enjoying it here?"

Jan's blue eyes remained dry, but his wavering voice and refusal to come near or meet Papa's eyes broke my heart. "I want to go home. The sisters are mean to Fritsje. They hurt him, and it makes me sad. Can we come home now? *Alstublieft*?"

"Come here, Jean-Jean. Papa wants to hug you."

Taking my brother's hand, I pulled him toward Papa. Then, slowly, slowly, Jan climbed onto Papa's lap and snuggled into his chest.

"I'm so sorry to hear all that, Jean-Jean. Tell me more," Papa whispered, his voice cracking.

Mama made an impatient sound. "Frits, you need to do as you're told when they tell you. Stop your belligerence. Look at how it upsets your *broertje* when you're punished!"

I opened my mouth to ask what "belligerence" means.

"And no talking back!"

Papa stared down at his hands and murmured. "I wish Toni and Jean-Jean could both come home, but Papa is still sick. That's why he's in this chair. Papa needs you both to be brave and stay here. It's for the best."

"Papa," I said thoughtfully. "Jean-Jean is a very good b…b…boy, but he's often scared. Maybe you could just take him…" I hated the idea of being at *het kindertehuis* on my own, but this was for Jean-Jean's sake.

"Sweet, sweet boy. *Nee*, Papa needs you both to stay here where you can be housed, fed, and educated." Papa took a deep breath and let it out slowly. "It's not what Papa wants, but he has no choice."

Planting my feet firmly, I furrowed my brow before bending to meet Papa's eyes. Maybe he didn't understand how determined I was. "It's okay. I don't mind not going to school…"

Doubtless fearing a meltdown was in the works, Mama interrupted by briskly getting to her feet. "Well, this has been a lovely visit, but now we must go. Frits, you'll probably have to take Jan out. Freddie, stop sniveling."

Papa's voice was weak, but he still objected. "Rita, let me kiss and hug them one more time. There may not be another. Then we can go."

I flung myself into my beloved father's arms. Now Papa's eyes did overflow.

Mama clenched her teeth, pulled Jan off his lap, and grabbed the wheelchair handles. "We're going, Frederik."

Gradually, as I stood at the playroom window with tears streaming down my cheeks, I became aware of a hand on my arm. It was Keetie.

"Come on, Fritsje. It's time for our lesson."

I smeared my hands over my face and mutely followed her. This was the routine now: on several evenings a week, Keetie patiently taught me to play the piano. Thus, we grew to be good friends. After a practice session, it was not unusual to see me leaning against Keetie, who was reading me a book while absent-mindedly stroking my hair.

Frits and Jan in the conservatory of *het kindertehuis* in Driebergen, 1938. (top)

The boys in the back garden on the day that they arrived, 1938. (bottom)

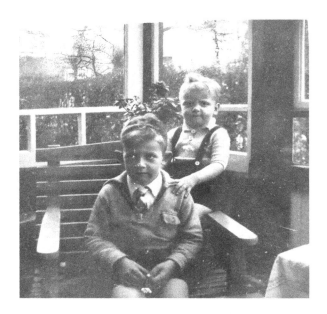

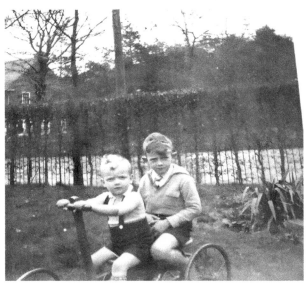

Children posing on a cart on Queen's Day, 1939. Frits can be seen almost at the back of the cart. Jantje is on the bench in the middle. Photo courtesy of Terry Brouwer. (top)

Zusters Deenik and Dermout, date unknown. (bottom)

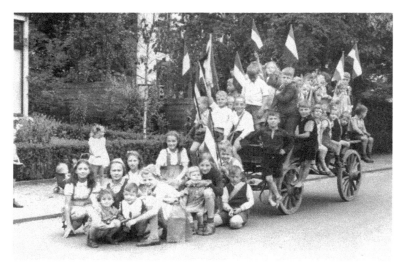

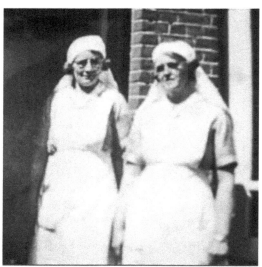

Mien Deenik en Suus Dermout

Frits and Jan with the de Viersprong dog, 1939. (top)

Zuster Deenik pulling a cartful of children with the help of a large dog, 1939. Jan is bottom right and Frits is top left. (bottom)

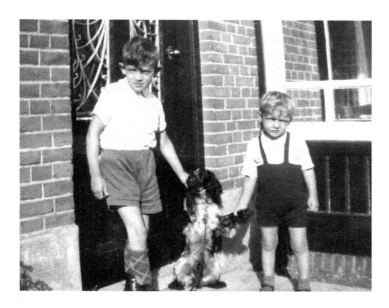

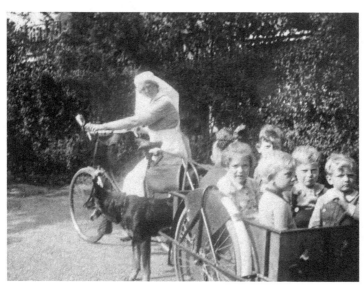

Keetie van Zanten just before she came to Driebergen. (top)

Jan is examining a newt in the forest in Driebergen while Frits looks on, 1940. Note Frits's black eye. (bottom)

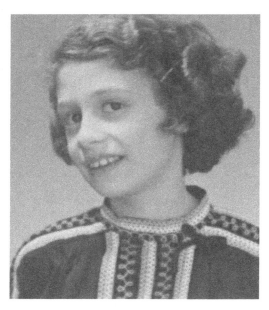

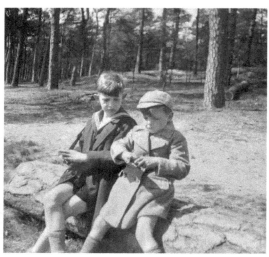

5

THE OCCUPATION

September 1939 brought three changes into my world, one good, one bad, and one that began as good but sure didn't stay that way.

First, I began attending the local school where Juf van Kempen taught my class. Whenever I arrived at school with a scraped knee or a black eye, she not only noticed but also gave first aid with her gentle hands. Fortunately, teachers at the Driebergen primary school on the Burgemeesterplein followed their class through the grades; Juf van Kempen was my teacher until I left Driebergen.

Second, World War II began. Juf van Kempen explained how, when Hitler invaded Poland, England and France declared war on Germany. The news had little effect on me. At six years old, I had no idea what war was. What I most feared, having our windows broken, didn't come to pass, so I figured we were safe.

Third, our maternal cousins came to live at *het kindertehuis*, bringing the total number of children in the home to 25, not counting Jantje.

"Edith, Meriam, I'm so glad you're here." With the sisters telling everyone what a difficult boy I was, it was a relief to have relatives who would be on my side, even if they were girls! Perhaps Edith would also help by easing Jan's loneliness; he was much too young for anyone else at *het kindertehuis* to befriend. His passive silence didn't help.

Meriam's mouth dropped open. "Wow! Frits, you speak Dutch!"

"Yup, I learned. No choice, really." I puffed out my chest.

Clutching Meriam's hand, three-year-old Edith's dark brown eyes swam with unshed tears, and her lower lip trembled. "I want Mama."

I had experience with this problem. After all, I'd been taking care of Jan for over a year now. Kneeling in front of the little girl, I took her hands in mine. "Edith, I know it seems scary here, but you'll have lots of fun. We go swimming in the summer; we take walks in *het bos,* sleep in bunk beds, and have yummy porridge for breakfast and dessert almost every day!"

Her little mouth formed a perfect O. "I love porridge!" she lisped.

Meriam giggled. "Now you know why Edith is the shape she is!"

"Mama says you're not allowed to make fun of me, Meriam! I look like her. Say sorry!" With her dimpled hands on her plump waist, Edith stamped her foot.

Meriam rolled her eyes before complying with her strong-willed sibling. "I'm sorry, Edith. Now, Fritsje, how is it here, really?"

"Well, let's sit over there so we can talk without the sisters overhearing us." I dropped my voice to a whisper. "First, tell me why your parents want you to live in Driebergen. Is one of them sick?"

Meriam's dark, wavy hair flew around her face as she shook her head. "*Nee,* they're fine. I think they're just worried, and Tante Aleida recommended this place to keep us safe."

I squinted my eyes. "Why wouldn't you be safe?"

"Because Herr Hitler hates *Joden.* Mama's friends wrote her that Hitler has camps all over Germany—and they're not good ones. *Joodse* people can't own businesses, and *Joodse* kids aren't allowed to attend school. In his Reichstag speech, believe it or not, Hitler said that if Germany goes to war, he wants to kill all of us! Every. Single. Jew. And they're at war now."

A chill went through me. Surely, all of that couldn't be true! I grasped desperately at a straw. "But, Meriam, we're not Germany. My teacher said the Netherlands is neutral about the war, and we're probably too small for Germany even to notice us. Surely, your family will be fine in Den Haag." Even as I spoke, my heart sank remembering the look in Juf van Kempen's eyes as she related the latest current events.

Meriam twisted a lock of hair between her fingers. "I hope so, but I overheard my parents and their friends saying they think Hitler might invade the Netherlands, anyway. Papa says he's a loose cannon."

"He's a cannon?" I frowned.

"That means they don't know what he'll do next."

I tapped on my lips as I thought this over. "So, why's your family staying? Why don't you all leave the country and go to England

70

or Canada? One of the *Joodse* shopkeepers in Driebergen did that just last month."

Meriam shrugged. "I'm not sure, but I think Papa and Mama hope that what they're worried about won't happen. They say they need to keep running their boarding house because they need the money. I doubt it since Mama's father has so much, being in diamonds. But they're supporting Tante Aleida now since the money Opa used to send her stopped. He died, you know. But she still has to be 'kept in the manner to which she has become accustomed.'"

I giggled at Meriam's imitation of our grandmother but had more questions.

"Opa died? And he used to provide for Tante Aleida?" Mama never spoke about her parents, especially her father, so I knew very little.

"Didn't you know? He used to send Tante Aleida some of the money he earned with his record deals. He was famous! The late great Henri Hartog Wallig. He died in Antwerp in May, and the funeral was huge. Mamma told me he killed himself because his German girlfriend was expecting his baby, and she married another man, a rich guy. Tante Aleida says that rumor isn't true, but then she would."

I grinned, enjoying my motor-mouthed cousin. "Oh, wow. How do you even remember all that? *Nee*, Mama didn't tell me. Not that she would! She doesn't stay long when she visits. But I still don't understand why Oom Henri and Tante Esther want you to live here. Is it safer here than in Den Haag?"

My cousin paused before answering. "Honestly, I don't know. But it was pretty stressful at home with Mama and Papa so worried, so I'm glad to be here with you! For them, maybe they think that if things get as bad for *Joden* here as has happened in Germany, they'll be able to react more quickly with Edith and me out of the way."

"Hmm, I wonder if that's why the other *Joodse* kids came, too."

"I wonder how many more we can expect."

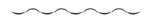

1940   Jan was now four years old, and my six-year-old self heaved a sigh of relief. He was the age I was when we moved to the Netherlands, and I knew that was big. The responsibility of caring for him no longer weighed on me quite as heavily. Therefore, when I saw Jan walk toward the garage while playing outside, I didn't follow him. Trouble and I were busy learning to roller skate with gadgets that we attached to the bottom of our shoes.

After he'd been out of sight for about 30 minutes, I noticed Jan return with a finger in his mouth and a frown on his face. I was pleased I'd been right not to worry but shook my head. I'd have to talk to him about sucking on his fingers; the older kids would make fun of him for sure.

That night, after lights out, Jan climbed up to the top bunk to snuggle with me.

"Jean-Jean, did you remember to put your pillow under the blanket in case the sister comes in to check if you're in bed?"

"Yup!"

"And you know that if someone comes in, you have to slide down under my covers fast?"

"Yup!"

"Okay then. Why are you here?"

"I hurt my finger today."

"Let me see." I examined the digit he offered and found a little blister at the end. "How did this happen?"

"I found a plug-hole in the garage wall and wanted to see if it still worked. Touching it made my hair stand on end, and my legs shake. And now my finger hurts."

Stifling my laughter, I kissed the offending finger. "Huh. I guess you won't do that again, you little scamp. Now get back into your own bed before you're caught."

From that day forward, I noticed that Jan always gave the broken copper electricity socket a wide berth—as if it would jump out and get him while he wasn't looking.

And I realized that perhaps four-year-olds aren't quite ready to be unsupervised.

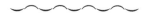

A week after my seventh birthday, Hitler attacked the Netherlands by bombing our entire coastline. I didn't notice. But, on May 14, when vast numbers of German bombers flew over Driebergen on their way to Rotterdam, I did. On May 17, with the surrender of Zealand, we officially became an occupied country. I later learned that many Jews committed suicide.

"Children, you'll have noticed German soldiers have arrived in Driebergen. They're here because our government surrendered to avoid more German bombs being dropped." Juf van Kempen's tone was carefully neutral.

I nodded. Just looking at the dapper soldiers with their shiny boots was utterly terrifying. Hearing the harsh sounds of the German language on our streets made my hair stand on end.

Marietta, one of the girls at *het kindertehuis*, waved her hand in the air. "Juffrouw, they're nice."

My teacher sighed. "I know. They do seem kind, but be careful. The soldiers act like that because many Dutch people have blue eyes and blond hair. Hitler considers us Aryan and hopes that, if they're friendly enough, we'll join his cause."

I looked around at the children in my class. Yup, mostly blond. Maybe we'd be safe. But then I noticed Keetie's, my cousins', and some of the other children's dark, shiny tresses. My heart sank. Not everyone was blond.

One of the village boys at the back of the class burst out, "Join him? Not likely, considering he bombed us! He killed my aunt, uncle, and all their *kinderen* when Rotterdam was demolished. My parents said they could drink his blood!"

Meriam joined in. "My mama told me Herr Hitler said he wants to exterminate all *Joden*—as if we're bugs! That's why they got fake IDs and will live in hiding with..."

Juf van Kempen silenced her with a look. "Those are good points, and honestly, the vast majority of Dutch people agree with you. But, now that we're occupied, keep those thoughts to yourself. It's for your safety. Also, the Germans have forbidden this kind of talk. Learn to bite your tongues!" Our teacher narrowed her eyes and looked at every child in the class to emphasize the warning.

"Juffrouw, are you saying that even here, far from the big cities, we're not safe?"

Juf van Kempen moved toward the troubled child and stroked her auburn hair. "I think we in Driebergen will be fine. After all, we're only six miles away from the headquarters of the National Socialist Movement (NSB) in Utrecht, and those Dutch men agree with Hitler. There's no reason for the German soldiers in our town to become aggressive. But...we're occupied by soldiers at war. Again, zip your lips!"

Trouble raised his hand. "Juffrouw, what about you? What do you think about Germany—are you an NSBer?"

I watched my teacher's cheeks flame and her eyes throw sparks before she carefully side-stepped the question. That told me more than she realized; she was not.

"We've talked enough. I'm not paid to talk about politics. My job is to teach you reading, writing, and arithmetic. So, open your math books to page 56."

We weren't done asking questions. Eddie's hand waved in the air. "But, Juffrouw, they're still fighting in Grebbeberg..."

"Math. Now." That was the end of that! Or so she believed.

I was still worried, and it looked like Trouble was also deep in thought.

Finally, school was over. I grabbed my coat and hat and rushed for the door. "Come on, Trouble, I'll race you home!"

"Hang on. I want to ask Juffrouw a question."

As I waited for Trouble, a blond, chubby-faced boy and a dark-haired girl walked over and joined me.

The boy grinned, making his freckles stand out even more. "Hi, Frits! I'm Herman Odewald, and this here is Rosalie Bloemist. Some of the village kids told us you guys live in a children's home, just like we do."

I paused a minute, thrown because he knew my name. "Yeah, we do. It's on the Arhemsebovenweg. But I didn't know there's another place like de Viersprong in Driebergen."

"Yup. Our home is on the Welgelegenlaan, not far from you. Well, Rosalie and I haven't been there long. The sisters only recently started taking in *Joodse* kids. Before that, the home was for asthmatics, but they all left. Now there's 11 *Joden.*"

Rosalie's sparkling eyes dimmed as she slammed her hand over Herman's mouth. "You're such a chatterbox. You're not supposed to tell anyone that, you know!"

"Oops! Don't tell, okay? We're pretending to be Gentile—we have new papers and everything." Herman attempted a wink.

Rosalie rolled her eyes.

I grinned and ran my finger across my lips. "I'll never tell. Cross my heart and hope to die." I looked over at Trouble. "Are you finally done? We'd better run to get back."

"Why?" Herman's eyebrows squished together, making his eyes turn into triangles.

"The sisters get mad if we're late. They may even beat me. Especially Zuster Dermout. One of the older kids told me she's a sadist. That means she's cruel, and she likes it!"

Herman's eyes became saucers. "Wow! The sisters who take care of us are really nice. Tante Bep and Tante To. I don't think either of them are sadists. But I'll ask."

"You're lucky. See you tomorrow!"

On the way home, Trouble and I chuckled as we imagined Tante Bep and To's reaction to being asked such a question. Even though I'd promised silence, we also discussed what I'd learned from Herman and Rosalie. After all, Trouble was my best friend. It seemed to us their caretakers were being overly cautious. But, what did we know?

Almost immediately after the occupation began, Jews were banned from air-raid shelters. By November, the authorities deprived Jewish professors, lawyers, and doctors of their jobs. Violence against Dutch Jews continued to increase with pogroms, forced deportation to labor camps, and random shootings. The Nazi gloves were off.

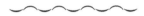

The snow was falling and the wind howling when Zuster Dermout grabbed my ear and pulled me to face her. "Frits, we're nearly out of wood."

"I'll go in a m…m…minute. I need to finish peeling potatoes first."

Zuster Dermout's backhand was quick, knocking me across my mouth. "You'll go now! Finish the potatoes later."

I hesitated. Leaving any job half-done made me very anxious, but her blazing eyes convinced me I'd better obey. Pulling on my threadbare coat and lining my boots, I slipped out the door while muttering about Zuster Gemenerik under my breath. I had no mittens, so I pulled my sleeves over my hands before grasping the wagon's metal handle.

Once in the nearby *bos*, I hastened to work, pushing snow aside to find sticks. The problem was that everyone else had also been collecting; very few were left. I moved deeper into the forest and smelled the campfire before I saw them.

Germans. Keeping my head down, I tried to creep to where they wouldn't see me. I'd heard rumors of random shootings, even in our little village.

Crraack! A stick broke under my foot.

"Hey, you there. Boy!" The guttural German accent rendered the soldier's Dutch almost unintelligible to my ears, but I stopped and looked up.

His booted feet planted wide apart, a flint-faced soldier with eyes that resembled chips of ice blocked my path.

"Y…y…yes, sir." I tried to keep my voice from shaking, but my efforts were to no avail. My stomach clenched so that I had to hold it with both hands.

"We need bread. Take this money, go to the baker, and buy a loaf. Bring it back here."

I glanced at the machine gun slung over the man's shoulder. Now, I faced a dilemma. Zuster Dermout would be angry with me for dawdling if I did as he asked. If I didn't, he might shoot me. Better to be disciplined. I took the money.

"Run! We're hungry."

Leaving the wagon behind, I took off as if a pack of wolves were on my tail, not stopping until I reached the baker. "Sir, I need a loaf of bread," I panted.

"Did Zuster Dermout send you?"

"No. I was collecting sticks in *het bos*, and a soldier gave me money to buy him bread." Because he and the sister were friendly, any lie would be discovered.

The baker crossed his arms over his chest. "Well, he's not getting any here. I'm not selling anything to *een vieze rot Mof* (a dirty rotten German)."

I felt like throwing up, so swallowed hard. "*Alstublieft*, sir. If I don't bring him bread, he might k…k…kill me!"

"Not if he can't find you…" The baker winked at me.

I knew what he was suggesting: I should take the money and return to *het kindertehuis*. But the sisters sent me to collect wood every day. That soldier would find me, no doubt about it. I had to take my chances with returning his money.

Blowing on my hands, I trudged back to the forest, where the soldier was waiting by my wagon. "Sir, I'm sorry, but the baker was all out of bread. Here's your money." I stood with my hand out, head down, and knees knocking. Would I now die? If so, I didn't want to see it coming. I shut my eyes tightly, just waiting.

"Oh. Thank you for coming back."

I glanced up at him in wordless astonishment before grabbing my wagon and pulling it to a part of the forest far from him. Fortunately, it was also far from where others had been gathering wood. Zuster

Dermout was so pleased with all the wood I found that she forgot to discipline me for being late.

Every year, on December 6, people in the Netherlands celebrate Sinterklaas, Saint Nicolas's birthday. Since the Nazis were determined that we be lulled into thinking nothing was going to change, this year was no different.

First, the stores brought out chocolate letters, Sinterklaas candy, and more, albeit less than usual and at inflated prices. At school, we sang Sinterklaas songs. Juf van Kempen talked about how Sinterklaas' servants, who all had the same name (Piet), were watching to see if children were good or bad.

I slumped in my chair. The sisters had convinced me: I was bad. On the rare occasions she visited us, Mama's lips often turned into a thin white line. I knew what that meant, too. There was little doubt in my mind that Jan would receive a *J* made of chocolate, *zuurtjes* (sour boiled candies), and a gift on the night before Sinterklaas, and I would be given a lump of coal.

"Fritsje!" Meriam stuck her elbow in my side just before dinner. "Why are you so glum? It's nearly Sinterklaas!"

I shook my head. "Everyone already knows I'm difficult. They only need to look at how often the sisters use the *mattenklopper* on me. But when even Piet doesn't bring me a gift…it'll just be embarrassing."

My cousin broke into peals of laughter. "Don't you know? Sinterklaas and the Piets aren't real. It's our parents who send the sisters money to get us stuff. I even saw where they have the chocolate letters." She stuck her elbow in my side. "Stop worrying! You'll get something."

"Really? How do you know?"

"Mama told me before we came here because I was worried Sinterklaas wouldn't know where we are. Trust me. The sisters will buy what your parents tell them to get for you."

"Are you sure?" This seemed a little too good to be true.

"Absolutely." Meriam gave a decisive nod.

"Oh, I hope I get a slide rule. I really want to learn how to use one."

This earned me an eye roll. "You're so weird!"

Chuckling, Trouble mimed wiping his brow. "Phew! Maybe I'll get something, too."

I hadn't realized he'd been listening to our conversation, but now I had my chance to play a trick I'd been planning for some time.

"I don't think so. People who tell lies get nothing, not even from their parents."

Under the table, I carefully colored the tip of my finger with a piece of chalk I had in my pocket.

Meriam gasped, and Trouble glowered at me. "I don't lie. What are you talking about?"

I pursed my lips and shrugged. "Ha! I have a foolproof way of knowing if you're telling the truth. You see, when you lie, your nose turns white." I touched his nose as I spoke. "I'll prove it. Tell me a lie."

Trouble crossed his eyes at me. "Um, you're a girl."

I turned to Meriam. "What color is his nose?"

Meriam giggled. "White."

"It is not! Edith, what color is my nose?"

Unfortunately, by now, our laughter had attracted Zuster Dermout's attention. "Dirk, you slovenly boy! You have chalk all over your nose. Go wash your face."

"Wash your face. Wash your face. Wash your face," Jantje echoed.

I grinned. The trick Papa once played on me worked perfectly.

That evening, with a much-relieved heart, I was happy to receive my gift, just like Trouble and the other children. It was a pair of socks, but it was a gift. Maybe I could wear them on my hands.

The best present came a week later: a letter from Papa. Just seeing his words made me feel warm all over.

Sweet Fritsje and Jean-Jean,

How are my sweet boys? Papa has been waiting for a letter from Fritsje for a long time, but it hasn't come. Mama told me you are working on a letter for Papa.

Did Sint Nicolaas come today, or did you see him at school? You need to tell me that. Did Piet scare your little brother, or was he okay? Did you sing lovely songs?

What a lot Papa wants to know, huh? Papa is already a lot better. Don't you think that's great, sweet boy of mine?

Give Jean-Jean a kiss from Papa and from Mama. Don't forget! And you also, I'm sending 100 XXXXX kisses.

How do you like Papa's writing? I tried so hard. Don't you think it looks as beautiful as your teacher's writing?

Goodbye. Paps

As was now my custom, upon finishing the letter, I held it to my face to inhale the lingering fragrance of Papa. Then, I continued to sit behind the curtains to think it over. What could I tell Papa about Sinterklaas? Socks were good, but they weren't a slide rule.

And why did Papa make a point of his handwriting? Papa was slurring his words the last time he visited, and I knew his sickness also made him weak. Could it be that, unlike what the letter claimed, he wasn't getting better? If not, why not?

My fears escalated. I remembered hearing about all the treatments Papa was receiving, but were they working? Or, worse, was he getting them?

When we complained about our empty stomachs and blamed the sisters, Juf van Kempen explained it wasn't their fault. She said that as soon as we became an occupied country, all food and fertilizer imports stopped, but food exports did not. The food shortage was exacerbated because the German soldiers ate much of what little was left.

Now I wondered, had imports of medicine also stopped? Was Papa even receiving the drugs he so desperately needed? The fragile thread of hope I'd been clinging to snapped, and I again felt the prick of tears behind my eyes.

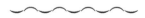

1941 Trouble threw his slate and chalk bag into the air. "Yay! We're free! No more school for six weeks!"

I laughed aloud but didn't follow suit. I knew I'd be unable to catch the slate, and Mama would be most unhappy if it broke. "Yup, we're going to swim and swim and swim!"

"First, we'll have to cycle the five km to the outdoor pool."

"Really? Do you think we're old enough not to go in the cart, even all the way to Woestduin in Doorn?"

Jan, who'd been tagging along, looked hopeful. "Maybe, since I'm still small, I won't have to go at all."

I rubbed his head. "Sorry, Jean-Jean, pretty sure they'll make you go."

Jan's shoulders rounded.

I could understand his feelings. Jan left the Congo before he was old enough to swim, but the sisters took their duty to teach him, without getting wet themselves, very seriously. They encased the poor child in a wide belt and hung him over the deep water with a thick fishing rod. By the end of last summer, Jan knew better than to scream but found it impossible to hold back his terrified whimpers. And he still remembered.

"Never mind. Maybe it'll rain," I suggested, noticing his pale face.

That night, I pondered Jan's predicament. I couldn't do much about his fear of water, but was determined that he should succeed in something. We began the next day.

"Come on, Jean-Jean, I know you can do it." I held the bicycle steady while my four-year-old brother climbed on.

"Okay, now, pedal!" I gave him a push and clapped as he wobbled down the street. Papa would've been proud, and I wished he could see his Jean-Jean.

"*Kinderen*, time to come in!" Zuster Dermout's jarring tones probably carried throughout the town.

Not having been taught how to brake, Jan fell off the bike. After picking him up and brushing him down, I stopped to watch the flood of children who were filing into *het kindertehuis*. So many! I'd been vaguely aware of more Jewish children coming to stay but now wondered just how many there were. Pointing at each one, I began counting.

"Frits! What are you doing? Dawdling again! Put the bikes away, then come in and get washed up for dinner."

Since we had to eat in silence, I counted while munching on one of my favorite meals: potatoes fried with a bit of onion. One, two, three… 34! Thirty-four children.

Deep in thought, I stopped chewing, put my knife and fork down, and rested my chin on my right hand. In January, Juf van Kempen told us anyone with a Jewish grandparent had to register as *Joods*. In February, we heard about a strike in Amsterdam protesting the harassment of Dutch Jews. I remembered her grimace as she later reported that it only took the German police a few days to suppress that action. Since then, the circumstances for Jews had only become worse.

What was happening at *het kindertehuis* was definitely odd, but I suspected that, like my aunt and uncle, other Jewish parents thought their children would be safe here. Obviously, the sisters were ignoring the recent German decree forbidding non-Jewish people from mixing with Jews. Could it be that those hard women had soft hearts?

Bang! My chin hit the table as my elbow was knocked out from under me. I swallowed the blood coming from my tongue before looking up at Zuster Gemenerik.

"No elbows on the table, Frits!"

Appie giggled, but Keetie gave me a sympathetic look. She knew better than to say anything.

I kicked at the fallen leaves, barely noticing the crisp smell of Fall. All was not well in my world. A week ago, I'd overheard Zuster Deenik telling Zuster Dermout that our town baker had been murdered—the one who'd refused to sell me bread. He was shuttering his shop windows a few minutes after curfew when soldiers shot him. Thinking of his body on the same flatbed truck where I'd seen soldiers throw everyone they killed made my stomach turn.

Yesterday, a couple of soldiers confiscated all the copper and bronze in *het kindertehuis*. That would mean less polishing for me, but their visit made me very nervous. Jan and I had a Jewish grandfather. And they might well have seen my cousins and Jewish friends. It seemed the sisters had the same thought.

At breakfast, Zuster Deenik tapped the shoulders of 16 children and instructed them to go upstairs as soon as they finished eating. I narrowed my eyes, noticing that Keetie, Meriam, Edith, and the other newer children were among those she singled out. All the Jews. I would really miss Keetie's infectious grin.

When the rest of us arrived at school that day, Juf van Kempen's eyes were suspiciously red. "*Kinderen*, I have to explain something very important to you—something that you must never ever repeat. Don't even talk about it amongst yourselves."

A hush fell over the room. Why was she even telling us?

"You'll have noticed that there are far fewer *kinderen* here than before. The *Joodse kinderen* won't be coming back to school since that's no longer allowed. But, and this is extremely important, you're not to talk about them with anyone. Remember always to say, '*Ik weet het niet*' (I don't know) in response to anything you're asked."

Wim's hand waved in the air. "Juffrouw, don't worry. Our *Joodse* kids are okay. It's just that the sisters told them to go upstairs this morning!"

One of the village boys snickered, but Juf van Kempen's face remained uncharacteristically solemn.

"*Nee,* they didn't. There are no *Joodse kinderen*. And, always, you saw nothing, and you know nothing. Remember that!" Our teacher looked around the room, making eye contact with each of her young charges.

From that day forward, the Jewish children didn't attend school. The third-floor curtains remained closed, and, well after dark, Juf van Kempen came and taught the children what they missed that day. If anyone knocked on the door during mealtimes, the Jewish children would scurry into the attic. They'd been well-trained.

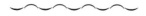

It was December again. Sinterklaas had come and gone with little jollity to mark the day. We sang the traditional songs and even put on a play, but behind closed doors. If no adults were present, we sang songs that had been altered to have lyrics about throwing bombs at *de Moffen*.

Sinterklaas was reported to have arrived in the country, but we all knew that rationing and the import ban meant candy and oranges wouldn't be available. After all, even food and soap were scarce by now.

If I was tempted to feel sad about the deprivation we were experiencing, another letter from Papa quickly cheered me up.

> Sweet Frits,
>
> What a beautiful letter you wrote! Papa and Mama were so happy with it, but we were even happier with your good report card. The sister is so pleased that she is going to give you two dimes! Papa will also put a dime in this letter, but I'm not telling you where. You will have to search for yourself!
>
> It's terrific that you had such a lovely presentation for Christmas. Be sure to tell Papa all about

it when you come to visit me in Den Haag because I really want to know how it went.

Goodbye Frits and Jean-Jean.

A *poempie* from Papa and Mama

It was always great to hear from my father, but it was even better to know Zuster Deenik had actually told my parents how well I was doing at school. I'd overheard Juf van Kempen tell Zuster Deenik how clever I was but figured my teacher was wrong. Everyone else just said I was difficult. Of course, the best news was that Jan and I were going to visit Papa. It would only be for a day, but I was counting down the minutes. Maybe he'd finally tell me what a "*poempie*" is!

Finally, the day arrived. Zuster Deenik accompanied Jan and me to the train station, paid our fare, and waited with us. "Alright now, Frits. Your mother said she'll be waiting for you in Den Haag. Just get off the train at that stop, and she'll be there."

Clutching Jan's hand to keep him safe on the platform, the wind whipped up my already wild hair. Mama would definitely frown on that, but there was little I could do about it. Butterflies were doing jumping jacks in my stomach as we climbed the steep stairs onto the train, but I smiled over my shoulder as if I had everything under control. "Of course, Zuster Deenik. We'll see you here again tonight."

Settling down in our seats, I unwrapped the piece of bread I'd snuck under my shirt during breakfast. I'd been much too nervous to eat. "Here, Jean-Jean, you can have this while we look outside. Maybe we'll see a snowman!" I couldn't point out cows and horses; they'd all been eaten.

The time until we reached our destination would have flown by if I hadn't been so petrified of the German soldiers sitting near us. I made sure never to make eye contact with them and kept Jan distracted by chattering about what I saw out the window.

It was a relief to see Mama standing on the platform, as promised. She gave each of us a brief air kiss before fastening Jan's hat more firmly on his head. "Whew, what a chilly day you chose. I'm glad the train was on time. Come on—it's not far."

I bit my lip as we trudged through snowdrifts to the tram. Since he'd been growing, it'd been hard to line Jan's shoes. I was used to the cold because I had to collect firewood every day, but he wasn't. Jan's nose was red, but there were no complaints, not even about his cramped toes, so that was a good sign. I figured that, for now at least, my responsibility to care for my *broer* had been satisfactorily discharged.

After the short tram ride, Mama turned and assessed us. Apparently, Jan passed muster, but I didn't. She pulled my collar higher and my sleeves lower. "We can't have you catching a chill and passing it on to Papa. I suppose you lost your hat? *Brr!* Let's hurry. The sooner we get there, the sooner we're warm."

I made no response, glad she hadn't noticed Jan was wearing my hat. He was the careless culprit, but I would never tell.

We plodded through unfamiliar streets in Scheveningen. Finally, Mama stopped by a snow-covered house that we also didn't recognize. "Papa is staying with his sister right now. Be sure to greet Oom Gerard and Tante Sophie loudly and clearly. His nurse may be there, too, but you don't need to greet her. She's just a servant."

Mama smoothed my wind-blown hair and again checked that our clothing was straight before she rang the doorbell. The door opened, and we were finally out of the bitter cold.

All the longings of the year since I'd seen my father welled up in me, and I pushed past Mama and Jan and ran up the stairs. Maybe I greeted my aunt and uncle, but I don't remember. I was totally focused on getting to Papa. Where was he? I scanned the room frantically, unable to bear another minute without him.

There he was, lying on the couch, his head on a thin pillow and his legs covered with a plaid blanket. His eyes were closed. I stopped stock still. How strange! Was he asleep...or worse? Even though I was no longer a little boy, I turned to grab Jan's hand before approaching.

"Hello, my dear sons," came a thready voice that I only just recognized. "Come closer. Kiss Papa—or are you too old for that now?"

I obediently bent down and kissed Papa's forehead before Jan did the same.

Papa struggled to open his eyes to a slit before catching one of our cold hands in each of his. "You can do better than that. Papa needs hugs—lots of them!"

Jan backed away, but I didn't need to be invited twice. I threw myself against the ailing man, drinking in his familiar scent and reveling in being near him. I wormed my arms under his frail body and squeezed as tight as I could. A strangled sound came from Papa's throat.

Mama quickly stepped forward. "Frits, be gentle. You're stronger than you think, and Papa needs to breathe."

I quickly released him, and Papa turned his eyes to Jan. "Don't you remember your very own Papa, Jean-Jean? Come here. Papa won't hurt you."

Jan put his finger in his mouth and stepped forward before slipping his hand into mine. His huge eyes were focused on the stranger lying on the sofa.

"Never mind. It's okay. Fritsje, can you help Papa sit up? Maybe with Mama's help. I want to feast my eyes on my sweet boys."

"Come on, Jean-Jean," I said. "You're strong. Let's show him—help pull."

A whisper of a grin formed on Jan's face, and between the three of us, we pulled Papa up and piled cushions behind him until he was close to sitting. Only then did Jan dare to move closer and allow himself to be surrounded by Papa's arm.

I perched on the side of the couch and told Papa the nice things about my life at *het kindertehuis*: my good grades, the swimming strokes I'd mastered, and beating my classmates in a bicycling race. I didn't worry him with the rest.

As I chattered, Papa's face lit up with pleasure. "I'm so glad to hear you're doing so well. But now, Mommy, I think it's time for the boys to unwrap their gifts. Can you get them, *alsjeblieft*?"

I could hardly believe my ears; my hands twirled in excitement. Mama told me that, with Papa sick, there was little money to spare. I hadn't expected to receive anything. After all, our toy cubbies at *het kindertehuis* were still empty.

My eyes shone as Mama placed two newspaper-wrapped parcels on Papa's lap. "Frits, you're the eldest, so you go first."

With trembling hands, I tore the paper off to reveal…skates! A brand-new pair of wooden skates with buckles so they could be tied onto boots or shoes. Entirely forgetting how fragile he was, I again threw myself at Papa. "Thank you, thank you, thank you! I can hardly wait to try these." I peered outside. The snow was still falling and the wind howling. It was looking good.

Papa's smile reached from ear to ear, and he messed up my hair. "Be sure and write to tell Papa how they work, okay? I need to hear from my dear boy."

I didn't answer, being far too busy examining the shiny buckles and sharp blades on my new skates even to notice what Jan received.

All too soon, our time with Papa had run out. He was again lying down, eyes nearly closed. "Toni, come here. I have something for you to remember Papa by."

He pressed an envelope into my hand, and I quickly opened it to find a photograph of him and Mama. "*Bedankt*, Papa. I'll put it up beside my bed."

"And Mama, *alsjeblieft,* take a photo of my boys and me so that I can remember them, too."

Mama got the camera; we stood by Papa, and she took the picture.

"Come now, boys. One last kiss for Papa, and you'll have to be on your way."

As I bent down to kiss his cheek, I was surprised to feel that it was wet. So was mine. Then I heard Papa whisper, "I'm so proud of you, Fritsje." I tucked those words deep into my heart, where they would have to last a lifetime.

On the way back to the train station, I told Mama about her nieces and how they were in hiding and now did their lessons in *het kindertehuis.* I figured talking would be safe because the weather had driven any lingering soldiers indoors.

"Yes, I already knew that. But you must be very careful not to speak about these things." She looked around anxiously.

I had pressing questions, so continued. "Yeah, my teacher already warned us. But Mama, Oom Henri and Tante Esther keep coming to see Meriam and Edith. Isn't that dangerous? Why do they do it?"

Mama's breath came out in a gust before she answered in a whisper. "You're right. It's not safe; my brother is an idiot. The Germans want all *Joden* to go to Amsterdam or a work camp, and things don't go well there. Your aunt and uncle are in hiding—or so I thought. Not that I know where…"

"I know, Mama! Since you got a job in Zeist and live there, they live in your house in Den Haag. Meriam told me. She and Esther even went to visit them."

Mama closed her eyes and shook her head. "Frits, don't tell anyone—you could get Mama in trouble! Poor Tante Esther and Oom Henri. I imagine they visited because they miss their girls so much." She continued under her breath. "And soon, there will be another to miss."

"What? What other one?"

"Did I say that out loud?" Mama shook her head before shrugging. "Well, you'll know soon enough. Your aunt is expecting a baby in the Spring. She thinks it's her duty to provide Oom Henri with a son."

I frowned. How did they know it would be a boy? Why would they miss the baby? Surely, they wouldn't have them live at *het kindertehuis,* too!

~~~~~~

1942

Dear Frits,

It has already been three weeks since you were with me, and I still haven't even heard if you arrived back safely in Driebergen. I expect it is very pretty in the forest with all the snow. Did you already make a snowman with eyes of coal and a pipe in his mouth? Is Jan still so frightened of the cold or not anymore? Does he join in with throwing snowballs? Is he still coughing so much?

Please write Papa a small letter. The sisters are so busy, and you are already so big that you can easily do it. You also need to tell me if you have tried the skates.

Goodbye, Frits, much love and a *poempie* for you and Jan-man.

Papa and Mama

Papa is getting much better and is even allowed to stand up in the afternoon. Wonderful, huh? Did you hang the picture of Papa and Mama up in your bedroom?

I am putting an envelope with stamps and paper in this letter. Give the sisters our greetings.

Goodbye, sweet boys.

Sitting in the corner of the playroom, I slowly lowered the letter to my lap. I felt so bad about not writing to Papa, but with all my chores, schoolwork, and skating, it was hard to remember to do it. *Nee*, that was an excuse.

Truthfully, I didn't know what to say. I wanted to explain that Jan was afraid of the cold and had a constant cough because the sisters made us exercise outside without shirts. That is unless it was snowing, in which case we had to do it in the kitchen in front of an open window. Every day. They said it was healthy, but I knew the houseboys would have disagreed.

I wanted to tell Papa all about how frightened I was lying in my bed listening for bombers. I knew *het kindertehuis* probably wasn't a target, but bombers often missed. Several houses in Driebergen had been obliterated. Would we be next?

I wanted to tell Papa that the sisters had an illegal radio hidden in a baby carriage. They called it "the baby," but I knew what it was because I'd looked. I was terrified that the Nazis would raid *het kindertehuis*, maybe because of the baby, or maybe because the sisters were hiding Jews, or maybe just because.

I wanted to beg my parents to let us come home, to tell Papa I'd be happy to take care of him, even if it meant never having time to do anything else. I felt guilty about enjoying my new skates, sledding, and running because I knew Papa couldn't. I ran my finger over the address at Maretakstraat 36. Was there even room for me there?

I wanted to pour out my aching heart and ask Papa if I was really as bad as the sisters said. I even wanted to tell him how hungry I was—and how taking care of Jan by sharing my food was forbidden. Surely, letting Jean-Jean go hungry was unforgivable.

I didn't have the words, so when I wrote, I said nothing of substance. And since the sisters didn't allow us to converse with them, my pain grew deeper and deeper until it was totally impossible to express.

Mama's answer was equally shallow. It pleased her and Papa that I wrote and didn't make too many spelling mistakes. When I read that she wouldn't be able to come to Driebergen until after Jan's birthday but wanted me to tell her what to bring when she did come, I put her letter down. How I wished she knew her sons well enough to know what they needed.

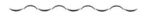

The curtains were closed in the playroom, and it was a hive of tranquil activity--sewing. Everyone who was female and old enough had a needle and thread in hand.

"Hey Keetie, what're you all doing?" Glad to be able to see her, I sidled over to where my friend was sitting, hunched over her sweater, sewing by candlelight.

"I'm obeying those *vieze rot Moffen*, sewing stars on my clothing, not that the sisters are letting us *Joden* go outside," she whispered.

"Can I help?"

Keetie's eyes crinkled. "Yes. Play something on the piano. It'll be great to listen, and it'll allow us to talk a bit without being overheard."

Over the next few days, as I walked to school and back, I noticed several people we passed had similar stars on their clothing. Juf van Kempen told us this was a new law—all Jews over six now had to wear stars with *'Jood'* written on them.

Questions arose in my mind. Why would the soldiers want Jews to be identified? My stomach turned over. Could it have something to do with Hitler's earlier proclamation about "exterminating" them? I'd seen enough violence to know that nobody was immune to the threat the Nazis posed. But surely this didn't include children!

Only a few weeks later, the sisters ordered all the Jewish children to stay upstairs on the darkened third floor—also during meals. They even slept there. If a nurse knocked on the wall, the children scurried up the pull-down ladder, through the hatch, and into the dark attic, where there was nothing. Not even a clock to help a person know that time was passing. I knew from experience that the only light was what seeped through the crack around the hatch. Although I missed sitting with my cousins and friends and didn't envy their seclusion, I was glad they were safe from extermination. For now.

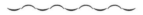

Early in June of 1942, Zuster Deenik came through the back door and into the kitchen, carefully carrying something in her arms. The sight of a tiny foot poking out of the blankets caused me to cease peeling potatoes and draw near.

"Ah Frits. You saw. This is your cousin. This is Hansje, Meriam and Edith's *kleine broertje* (little brother)."

She pulled back the blanket. There, in her arms, was a round pink baby with startlingly blue eyes. He was so beautiful that I caught my breath.

Zuster Deenik, evidently gentled by the cooing infant, smiled. "You can touch him, you know."

I quickly returned to the sink, washed my hands three times, and reached out. After stroking his shiny blond hair, I slipped my finger into his little fist. How could something this small even be a person?

"Do you want to hold him? I think, now you're nine, you can do it. But be careful—he's only a month old!" Zuster Deenik indicated that I should sit on the kitchen stool.

"Be careful to support his head," she warned before placing the warm, sweet-smelling bundle into my arms. Unable to resist, I bent over and kissed Hansje's cheek. I was unaware of the pearls raining down my cheeks until they dripped onto his forehead in a baptism of love.

Zuster Deenik removed her coat and slipped on her apron before taking him back. "I'd better introduce him to his sisters now."

Finally, my words returned, and I dared to ask a question. "Will he be living here?"

"Of course. Where else? We just need to be very careful that he isn't too loud."

"Won't his mama miss…" My voice tailed off as Zuster Deenik swept out of the room. Evidently, that didn't matter. I didn't need to ask why. Hansje was the newest *onderduiker* (person in hiding) in *het kindertehuis*.

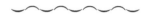

"Frits, you have a letter."

I slid off my chair and took the envelope from Zuster Deenik's hand. The address was in Mama's handwriting, but the return address said she was living at the Prins Mauritslaan 67. That was strange, but I guessed it was because there was no room with Papa, and my aunt and uncle were renting Mama's house in the Bezuidenhout.

I took a deep breath before beginning to read.

Dear Fritsje and Jean-Jean,

I'm coming again to Driebergen on Sunday. Good, huh? I'm looking forward to seeing you both.

Why haven't you written, Fritsje? I've been very busy, so can't write frequently, but that's why I'd like to hear from you. Didn't you even think about that? Now you don't need to since I'm coming on Sunday, but after that, you really need to write. Also, to Papa.

You didn't even write Papa to thank him for the skates that you got for your birthday! But you should have. I thanked him for you, but he deserves to hear from his son. I'm determined that he will.

Say hi to the sisters and lots of kisses for Jean-Jean.

Papa and Mama

"What did she say, Frits?" Jan pulled on my arm.

"Nothing, except she's coming on Sunday. And she's mad at me again."

Jan's face fell. "Never mind. Come on! The horse and cart are waiting."

Today, those children who weren't in hiding would go to the Pyramid of Austerlitz, giving the impression of life as usual. The sisters bustled around, gathering picnic supplies and ensuring everyone looked tidy before they stepped into the wagon.

On the way, Juf van Kempen, who'd come along for the ride, quizzed us.

"Who knows who built the pyramid and how old it is?"

Marietta's hand waved in the air. "A French general made his troops build it because they were bored."

There was a titter, and Marietta looked daggers at the offender before insisting. "It's true! And it's been there since 1804."

"So, how old is it?"

That was a little more difficult, but I loved math. "138 years, give or take a few months."

Juf van Kempen's smile made me puff up my chest. "Yes, very good. And who wants to go to the top of the obelisk?"

I put my hand in the air and glanced at Jan. His was the only hand not waving. He hated heights.

"You'll be okay, Jean-Jean. I'll be with you. And afterward, we can learn about what it was like in the Netherlands during the French era."

Jan looked up, hopefully. "And go to the playground, right?"

"Yup, of course." I wanted to see Jan smile, but that was a thing of the past. By now, smiles were rare. Very rare.

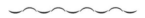

The sun was shining, but the world was gray. It felt like we'd been occupied forever. Juf van Kempen told us that an NSBer had replaced the mayor of Utrecht. Naturally, this gave the Germans license to carry out more atrocities, not that they needed permission. Raids and on-street violence became commonplace, rendering daily life terrifying.

While waiting in line to buy potatoes, my attention was caught by a conversation between two elderly women standing in front of me.

"Have you noticed how few stars we now see on the street? It seems the *Joodse* population are going into hiding," said the black-clad woman with a gentle face.

"It won't help," cackled her companion. "They'll be caught."

"Do you think so? I've heard that conditions in the ghetto in Amsterdam are terrible. Many families crowded into one room, broken plumbing, rampant disease, and very little food. People are dying there, Agatha!"

"Serves them right, those greedy capitalists. See if they think they're "chosen" now!" Agatha crossed her arms over her bony chest. "I hope all the *onderduikers* are caught! Death is too good for scum like that. I'm sure you agree, Maaike."

Temporarily abandoning my quest for potatoes, I quickly slipped out of sight behind a shelf but peeked around the corner and continued to listen.

Maaike adjusted the scarf over her head, but I could see that her blue eyes had become like saucers. "Oh, my! But…"

"*Ja*, if I hear of anyone hiding *Joden*, I'll report them. They can join the animals they love so much—in Buchenwald, Mauthausen, and Auschwitz."

"Um, well, oh my. Oh, it's your turn to be served, Agatha."

Before Agatha spoke to the greengrocer, she pierced Maaike with narrowed eyes. "I'm sure you agree with me, don't you? Answer me!"

"Oh, *ja zeker*. Of course."

But when Agatha turned away, Maaike's shoulders grew even rounder.

I waited until both women were gone before rejoining the line, but it was no use. The potatoes were sold out. Walking home with my arms wrapped around my waist, I thought about the *onderduikers* I knew and loved. I never saw Meriam, Edith, and Keetie and only rarely heard little Hansje crying. Did they feel sad up there on the third floor? They had to be so quiet! Their curtains were permanently closed, and lights were forbidden. Were they even allowed to look outside and see the trees and sky? How could I help?

Suddenly, I realized. As Keetie originally suggested, while she was sewing on her star, I could both cheer them up and cover any noise they made. Maybe even a conversation among themselves. Once I got back, I opened the book from which Keetie had been teaching me and played the piano. Loudly. The mistakes didn't matter since my goal was to drown out any noise from upstairs. Surely, they would figure out what I was doing!

In no time, I found myself enjoying the music, even swaying as my fingers pounded out the notes. A group of children gathered around and sang those songs that had words. Trouble played drums on the table while Wim kept time with a baby's rattle.

The cacophony attracted Zuster Deenik, who came in frowning but soon forgot to be worried about her colleague's reaction. We all needed cheering up. It wasn't easy to hold back my chuckles when she joined us in singing, sounding much like a bullfrog.

Eventually, even Zuster Dermout joined her caterwauling voice to ours. The sound was certainly not beautiful, but it sure felt good.

That night, my old friend panic once again assaulted me. Thinking about what might happen in the future, especially if the Nazis discovered the Jewish children, my stomach clenched, and my breath sped up. Unable to get comfortable, I decided to risk the sisters' wrath. I snuck upstairs and felt my way to what I hoped was Meriam's bed.

"Hey, Meriam, are you awake?"

"Frits?" Sleepy eyes peered at me through the gloom. "Well, I am now." My cousin sat up, pushing back her tangled hair.

"Come on. Let's t…t…talk. I miss you!"

"What if the sisters catch us?" Meriam whispered.

"Who cares? Come on!"

She didn't need to be invited again. Sharing her blanket, we huddled together in the stairwell. "Tell me, how are you doing? Aren't you sad hiding up there? Do you ever hear from your parents?"

Meriam pulled the blanket closer around her thin shoulders. "I'm okay. Kind of." She shrugged. "It's not as if any of us have a choice in this. After all, the Nazis are always watching. Mama sometimes writes—she's in hiding now too, you know."

I opened my mouth to tell her I knew where they were and that they still went out to parties but closed it quickly. Mama told me not to tell anyone what she'd shared in a moment of frustration.

Meriam continued, "A friend delivers the letters, and the sisters bring them up when nobody is looking."

I pillowed my chin on my hand. "Couldn't your father visit you, or does he wear a yellow star?" I knew he was my mama's brother, and she didn't wear a star. So maybe…

"Why, of course he does! He has to, and he's in hiding, too. What a strange question! Why did you ask?"

"Oh, I think I hear someone coming! I better go." I flew down the stairs while Meriam disappeared into her room.

I wondered why Mama didn't wear a star but was sure that the fewer people who knew of her mixed heritage, the better. I could perhaps ask Papa, but his last visit to us had been canceled. Although his letters said he was getting better, my heart knew differently. His time was running out.

It was the last day of the semester, and we crowded around the board to find out if we'd passed our exams.

"Hey, Frits, you toad! You came top of the class in history and math!" Trouble punched me in the arm.

"Hmm, well, you couldn't have come far beneath, considering you're always copying my work."

"*Ja, ja*. As if anyone would believe that. We all know why you did well: I taught you everything."

"You're crazy. That makes no sense! Anyway, we're free! Let's go for a bike ride through *het bos*."

In no time, a group of children had mounted their bikes and were cycling through the woods with the wind in their hair.

"Bet you can't cycle up and down the Swiss Bridge!"

"Ha! Just watch me!"

Just then, I noticed Jan standing at the bottom of the wooden bridge, looking up while biting his lip. It was very high. Unfortunately, I wasn't the only one who noticed his hesitation.

"Hey, look at the little coward!" Hans, who should have known better, jeered at my brother.

"Take that back!" Even though he was bigger than me, I flew at him, fists clenched. I only got in one punch before he recanted his words, but the damage was done. I saw Jan's face.

"Come on, Jean-Jean. Let's go catch a newt at the Koekenpan pond."

"Maybe we could set a fire, too."

I frowned at my little brother. Sometimes, he baffled me. "Well, I guess. But we'll have to put it out before we're caught."

Jan nodded. But he didn't smile.

Fortunately, that day, the German soldiers seemed to be engaged elsewhere. I saw nothing to rob me of my joy that the summer vacation was starting. But, all too soon, something would.

Frits and Jan visiting Papa, 1939. The photograph from the later visit has been lost. (top)

Children in a tree at *het kindertehuis*. Frits is on the right and Meriam is next to him, 1941. (bottom)

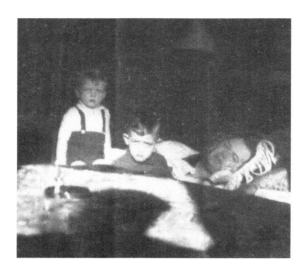

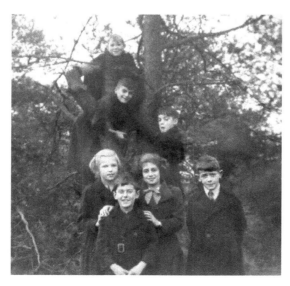

Frits at school, September, 1941. (top)
Letter from Papa, December, 1941. (bottom)

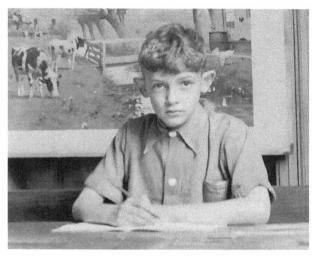

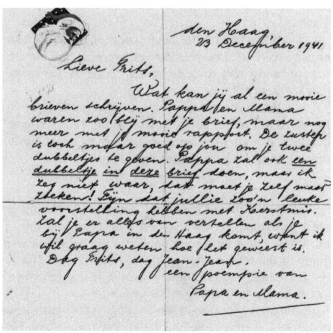

6

THE BEREAVEMENTS

July 22, 1942

Dear Frits,

So, my son, you passed. How wonderful, huh? Papa is so happy about that, and Mama will be too when I tell her. She is in Amsterdam right now, taking a few days of vacation. When she comes back, I'll quickly show her your letter. I also saw that your grades are good.

When will you have vacation, or did you already have it? The weather isn't so nice now, much too cold and yucky to go swimming. You love to swim, don't you, Frits?

When you come to Papa, bring your diploma so I can see it. I'm not doing so well again. I miss you so much, and your little brother. Goodbye, sweet boys; much love and a lot of kisses from Papa.

Goodbye

Scowling, I read and reread this letter while tracing my finger over the last paragraph. It was the first time Papa told me he wasn't doing well. I now knew he'd been unable to get his medications since the beginning of the war, so he was bound to get worse. But it worried me that he was actually admitting it. Why did he say "goodbye" twice? I quickly penned a response, hoping to find out more.

Unfortunately, because of the time taken for wartime mail to be delivered, before I even received his letter, Papa was gone. He died on July 26 at his sister's home in Rotterdam while Mama was still in Amsterdam. He never saw my carefully penned and loving answer.

Mama came to Driebergen on August 16 and told us about Papa's death. By then, he'd already been buried. My heart broke into pieces, and the shards rendered it almost impossible to breathe. Jumping up, I ran from the playroom and out the back door of *het kindertehuis*. I didn't return until I saw her leave.

Overwhelming desolation found its way into a veritable flood of tears. I was drowning and neither uttered a word nor smiled for the next two weeks.

Zuster Deenik came to stand next to me as I again pushed away my dinner plate. Even though refusal to finish every mouthful would usually result in a beating, my grief stayed her hand and carved a line between her eyebrows. I saw little reason to eat, and the thought of doing so made me gag. Papa was the only person in the world who totally understood me, who accepted and loved me, who thought I was amazing just because I was me. He called me Toni because he wanted me and thought me to be beyond praise.

I obsessed over the fact that Mama never wanted children, whereas Papa stood on his head for joy about me. The pain of my loss was overwhelming. I refused to do my chores, almost daring the sisters to beat me. At least then, I'd feel something. I ignored Jan's silence, even though I figured he was suffering, too. There was no color in my world, and I had nothing left to give.

"Frits and Jan. Letter for you both."

With dragging feet, I plodded forward. Zuster Deenik's hand lingered on mine as I listlessly accepted the letter.

Mama's handwriting was on the front. Of course. The sisters had recently bought and sent her birthday gifts on our behalf. Had she received them in time for her birthday on August 23? I didn't care. But maybe she'd write something about Papa's last days, even though she hadn't been there. I hungered for anything.

Den Haag, 8/24/42

My dear boys,

Thank you very much for your beautiful gifts for my birthday. The parcel arrived very nicely on time. I am thrilled with that brush hanger. I just needed it so much because my clothes brush was always lying in a corner, and that really shouldn't be. I immediately hung the hanger and put the brush in it. It looks so tidy!

I am also delighted with the birthday calendar. I also needed it very much because remembering birthdays is not my strong suit. Now I won't forget people. I've already filled in several birthdays. You're on it, too, even though I wouldn't forget you!

The letter stand is a bit wobbly. I will have to receive a lot of letters before they are fixed in it, so write, Fritsje, often.

How nice that you had such a good time, and how much you will have enjoyed that driving tour! And you have also been on the watchtower, I heard. Uncle Hans certainly wasn't afraid, was he? But I didn't like it at all, remember? Was it a nice view at the top, and has your brother been that high?

I was very sorry that you were not here yesterday on my birthday. In any case, you will soon come and stay for a few days, then we will also go out, maybe to the zoo. Would you like that? I'll write to you as soon as I can!

Good day, dear boys!

Lots of kisses from Mama.

I folded the letter and slipped it back into its envelope. It seemed like Mama had forgotten about Papa. I didn't understand how she could summon the energy to be excited about a brush hanger. Could it be that Mama expected us to move on as if Papa had never existed? I took a deep breath. Being miserable wouldn't bring him back, so maybe she was right. From then on, even though I nearly choked on it, I stuffed the pain down deep and pretended to be okay. Maybe, one day, I would be.

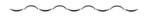

September marked an important event in Jan's life: he was now old enough to attend the village school on the Burgemeesterplein. He was too big at six to hold my hand, but as we walked to school, his little body pressed so close to mine that walking was not easy.

"It'll be okay, Jean-Jean. Maybe your teacher will be as nice as mine. And remember, there's no school on Sundays, Saturday afternoons, and Wednesday afternoons. We can do something fun on all those days."

Anxiety over my brother plagued me all day. How was he doing? Had he made friends despite being shy? I bolted out of the door the moment my class was dismissed. There he was, pressed against the building as if trying to disappear into the brickwork.

"How was it, Jean-Jean? Did you love it?"

Jan shook his head and muttered. "I hated it. The village kids are mean. They told me we from de Viersprong are intruders into their school."

Although my hands involuntarily formed into fists, I kept my face bland. "Give them time. Some are my friends—well, kind of. And if they see you're nice…"

Jan stopped short to glare at me, his eyes spitting sparks of fury. "*Nee,* they'll never like me. Nobody does. And my teacher is horrible, too. She doesn't care what they say or if I do any work. I spent the whole day watching the flies on the windows."

"Well, tomorrow might be better. You never know."

The next day, whenever I remembered, I crossed my fingers on both hands. It didn't help. Jan hated school the entire time he was in Driebergen, and, as far as I know, he didn't learn a thing. There were murmurs about dyslexia, but he was right. His teacher didn't care.

A few days later, I was doing a crossword when I heard ear-splitting shrieks coming from the kitchen. Jan! Zuster Deenik jumped to her feet and ran, but I got there first. My dry-eyed but very loud brother was standing with a pencil in one hand and blood dripping from the other.

Zuster Deenik grabbed the sodden appendage and bent over his hand to search for the source of the blood. "Stop that noise. Then tell me what happened."

Jan took a deep breath and told what I was sure, based on the evidence, was a whopper. "I…I…I caught my finger on the fence."

I was going to need to talk to him about his lying skills. After all, he was in the kitchen with a pencil in his hand, not outside! I cast my eyes around the stool he was standing by. Yup. There on the floor was a sharp knife.

Distracted by the fact that he'd cut one nail entirely in half, Zuster Deenik grabbed a cloth, wrapped the hand, and loaded him into the cart at the back of her bike. Left behind, I quickly hid the evidence that would land him in hot water.

My silly little brother, trying to sharpen his pencil with a kitchen knife! Since the sisters didn't permit questions, this type of ingenuity was inevitable. I would show him the right way to sharpen pencils when he returned.

When Jan returned, however, he was in no shape to learn anything, neither about lying nor about sharpening pencils. Dokter Hermans had treated his injury by pulling off the entire nail! For the first week, moans of pain punctuated every night.

"Just wait until I tell Mama what that nasty *dokter* did!"

"Um, little guy, remember when we saw her in August? She said she wouldn't be back until after Christmas. It'll be better by then."

It was several weeks before Jan could even pick a pencil up, and his finger was deformed for the rest of his life. Not that Mama noticed.

Sinterklaas and Christmas came and went without special attention. The shops had nothing to sell, and neither Jan nor I received a gift from Mama. I didn't care since I was just going through the motions of life: getting up, dressing, going to school, coming back, doing chores, and going to bed. Even riding a bike through the forest no longer brought me pleasure. Stuffing my feelings made me numb not happy. I was nine, but felt like 90.

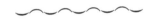

1943 While sitting at the table, supposedly doing math, I observed that the Zusters Dermout and Deenik were deep in conversation. Without lifting my head, I strained to hear.

"What can we do? Our supplies are so low. We don't have enough to feed, or even wash, *de kinderen.*"

"We could always use our rations for them…"

"Ration books don't help when the shops are empty." Zuster Deenik's shoulders were stooped, and she clasped her hands over her waist.

Zuster Dermout patted her on the shoulder. "Don't worry. I don't think it'll get much worse for us. You know how Meneer Tonnon was appointed to replace Burgemeester (Mayor) de Beaufort?"

"*Ja*, and?"

"Well, Tonnon is my brother's best friend. And, as a long-time NSBer, he has access to stores that others don't."

"Do you think he'll help us? We're a children's home, and what he has belongs to the Germans."

"Of course, he will. He wants to gain favor with the town, and this is a good way to do it." Zuster Dermout chuckled without humor.

"Actually, he tries to please everyone: the Germans, the bourgeoisie, and the NSB. We can use his weakness and, frankly, cowardice to our advantage."

I jumped up; my fists clenched in anger. How could the sisters even think to have anything to do with a German collaborator?

Zuster Dermout noticed my movement and, grabbing Zuster Deenik's arm, steered her out of the room.

Sinking back into my chair, I pillowed my chin on my hand. What could I do about this? It seemed our meals would be provided by NSBers, people who helped those who deprived my papa of the medicine he needed. Since I knew it, would eating make me a traitor, too? I could refuse the food, but the sisters never let us leave anything on our plates. Just one more thing to feel guilty about.

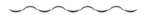

Being engrossed in a book that explained how radios work, I jumped at the sound of the doorbell. Who could that be? It was too late for parental visits.

Zuster Deenik pushed herself out of her chair and lumbered stiffly toward the front door. Curious, I peeked around the corner of the playroom down the hall. She opened the door to reveal a swarthy, slender man with a bushy mustache. He appeared to be in his late 20s. Beside him was an equally dark-haired and skinny woman who looked slightly older.

"Hello? Can I help you?" Zuster Deenik kept her hand on the door.

The woman wrung her hands and spoke with a thick German accent. "We're sorry to disturb you, Zuster. I'm Anni Amalie, and this is my brother, Siegbert Werner Flatow. We just arrived in Driebergen and met Zuster Dermout on the Traaij. She was so friendly—unlike many of the villagers—and invited us to stop by anytime. So here we are."

"I see." Zuster Deenik looked over her shoulder. "I know you're there, Frits. Go get Zuster Dermout."

I mounted the stairs to tell Zuster Dermout about our visitors and then stood at the top to see what happened next. Why would Germans visit us? This was more entertaining than the entire day had been.

103

Zuster Dermout squeezed past me and sailed down the stairs with her hands extended. "So good to see you both, Meneer and Juffrouw Flatow. Come in. Let's have a cup of tea."

Zuster Deenik, shaking her head in confusion, followed the pair into the living room while Zuster Dermout hurried to give orders to the kitchen staff.

Once they were all settled in the living room, the door was closed, and the show was over. There they remained until it was time for our bath and bed.

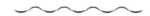

"Frits!" Jan's voice woke me from a deep sleep.

"What?"

"I have to pee."

"You know that's not allowed. You shouldn't have drunk so much water. Just hold it until morning."

"I can't!" My brother's voice rose to a whine.

"Well, use the sink in the hallway. That's what I do. But be quiet so you don't get caught."

"I can't reach that high."

I sighed and turned over to go back to sleep. "Don't know what to tell you."

In the morning, I remembered Jan's predicament and asked him how the night had passed. I hoped he hadn't wet the bed since that brought severe punishment down on the offender's head.

"I had to go bad, really bad, Frits."

I rolled my eyes. "Yeah, I know. So, what did you do?"

"I went."

I jumped out of bed. "Did you wet…"

Jan's eyes sparkled, and his grin lit his face. "Nope." Then he pointed out the door of the bedroom.

Our conversation caught Trouble's attention. He smirked and followed where Jan was pointing with his eyes. "You're kidding!"

Now on the landing, I called back in. "He's not."

To explain, just outside the green bedroom, on the landing, was a large white cupboard with two doors and two drawers. The sisters stored the linens: sheets, towels, pillowcases there. They'd also filled the bottom two drawers with sheets and, last night, must have left one of them slightly open. Jan just made use of the crack. No one ever noticed; at least nobody said anything.

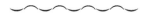

The next night, I was again awoken, this time by Meriam, who was wrapped in her blanket and standing by my bed. "Uh, Meriam, what are you doing down here?"

"Come upstairs—quietly! I need to talk with you."

I grabbed my sweater to put on over my pajamas. It was nearly December, and the windows were open since the sisters believed in fresh air. Together, we crept into the stairwell, where Meriam sank down and buried her face in her hands.

I patted her shoulder awkwardly. "Are you sick? Should I get Zuster Deenik?"

"No! Oh, I'm so scared! I hate being up here!"

I knit my brows and scratched my head. "Not really sure what you're talking about. I know hiding stinks, but you're safe up here. Well, as long as a bomb doesn't fall on us."

Meriam shook her head. "We're not safe. Not at all."

"Why do you say that? Nobody knows you're here. At least no one who would tell…"

Gripping my hand so hard that it hurt, Meriam whispered, "You know how we used to meet kids in *het bos* who live at the children's home on Welgelegenlaan 29?"

I was confused by this change of topic, but I went with it. "*Jawel*. Trouble and I used to play with Herman and Rosalie. Well, until they stopped coming to school. They always said their nurses are kind. I kind of wished my mom sent us there."

"*Nee,* you don't! Listen! Apparently, the kids who were there are all *Joden*, but the nurses gave them non-Jewish names and papers so nobody would know."

"*Ja,* I knew that. Herman told me. Wait! Were there? Where are they now?"

Meriam took a deep breath and placed trembling fingers against her lips. "They were betrayed."

"What?" A chill went through me.

"Zuster Dermout told us yesterday, but it happened last week. She warned us to stay extra quiet because of it. Apparently, lots of people saw an armored car with German intelligence officers drive up to the front door of Welgelegenlaan 29. They took the two nurses and ten *kinderen* to the train station. I guess the train went to the ghetto in Amsterdam since that's where they take *Joden*."

"Umm, pretty sure 11 kids were living there."

"There were. But Jack's parents moved him somewhere else just last month. Lucky kid!"

"Well," I said doubtfully, "Maybe Amsterdam isn't so bad?"

Meriam shook her head. "You know it is but *Joden* don't stay there. The sisters said *de kinderen* were almost immediately moved to Weteringschans and then Westerbork. I guess Zuster Dermout's brother told her. The next stop is probably Auschwitz. My parents told me that's a terrible place." She wrapped her arms around her belly and rocked back and forth, her eyes staring sightlessly.

"Herman and Rosalie, too?" I hoped perhaps my friends had been overlooked.

"All the kids."

"Tante Bep and Tante To?" I asked in a strangled whisper.

"Kamp Vught, a concentration camp."

I reached out for Meriam, and we sat enfolded in each other's arms until I heard the clock chime 3:00 am.

"We'd better go to bed. Hopefully, you're worried about nothing. After all, those kids weren't hiding. You are."

Meriam's sigh came from the bottom of her soul.

I watched my cousin in her white nightgown slowly ascend the stairs, her dark head bowed, before creeping to my bed.

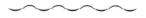

Dinner consisted of sugar beets mashed with a potato or two. Distinctly disagreeable, but I dug in. Hunger makes almost anything taste good. Not that. But almost anything else.

Just then, the back door opened, letting in a gust of wind. I glanced at the window. It was pitch dark outside, much too late for Juf Flatow's usual visits.

The playroom door flew open even before Zuster Deenik put her knitting aside and laboriously got to her feet, presumably to see who had let themselves in.

Juf Flatow, with reddened eyes and windswept hair, hurried to meet her. "Oh, Zuster Deenik, the most terrible thing just happened."

"Sit down, Anni. Tell me." Zuster Deenik waited while Juf Flatow took off her snow-covered coat and then grasped Anni's trembling hands.

"It's Siegbert. He's such an idiot! He was smuggling black-market cigars. You know we had to make a living somehow. It's not as if anyone would give a German and a Jew a job! Well, they caught him. He's been arrested!"

Zuster Dermout joined the other women, pursed her lips, and shook her head. "So foolish. What can I say?"

Anni covered her face and wailed, "Oh, what can I do? He's my little brother!"

"Nothing. It's not up to you now. He's not a child. Go home and pray." Zuster Dermout folded her arms across her chest.

"I'm so worried that I feel sick." Anni hiccupped, "Can I stay here for a little while?"

Zuster Deenik opened her mouth, but Zuster Dermout interrupted. "No. Absolutely not. Frankly, I'm worried your frequent visits have already drawn the attention of the Nazis. This ridiculous behavior of Siegbert's will make it worse. *Alsjeblieft,* don't come again."

My mouth dropped open. Those words were very harsh. But, on the other hand, she had a point.

Juf Flatow looked at Zuster Deenik, perhaps hoping for a different verdict. Pressing her lips together, Zuster Deenik shook her head and pointed to the door.

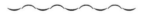

1944 It was January 6. That day, we went to school as usual, but before it was even lunchtime, Juf van Kempen told us we were to go back to *het kindertehuis*. Immediately. No dawdling.

Despite our ages, I gripped Jan's hand. My stomach hurt, and my mouth was dry.

"*Kinderen,* take off your coats and go straight into the playroom." Zuster Dermout's tone was even higher and tighter than usual. Our shoes clattered, but our voices were uncharacteristically silent.

Zuster Dermout held the door open while we filed in. Even though Jan and I were at the back of the queue, I could see that the big table had been moved out of our line of sight. The chairs were stacked up on one wall.

When we reached the doorway, I stopped short. There, behind the long wooden table, which was now in front of the rain-streaked window, sat two Nazi officers, their insignia gleaming. Next to them was a Dutch man without a uniform, doubtless an NSBer. In front of them was a card index.

"Go on in, boys," said Zuster Deenik, pushing me from behind. Then she raised her voice. "Everyone, wait for me here. I'm just going to get the *Joodse kinderen*."

Total silence reigned in the playroom. I put my arm around Jan's shoulders while Zuster Deenik ran upstairs to order the frightened young *onderduikers* from where they were hiding in the attic. They shuffled in, heads down. Meriam's face was white, her lips moving in a silent prayer. When Keetie glanced at me, I saw that the sparkle usually present in her eyes had fled.

My forehead wrinkled while we waited for what was next. The Jewish children had been kept hidden for months but had now been dragged to a ground-floor room with an enormous window. In front of Nazis! This could not be good. I drew Jan to the back of the group of terrified children, where the plastered wall breathed its cold into our small bodies.

Glancing up, I caught my breath at the emptiness in the NSBer's eyes as he read out the instructions. "Everyone, stand on the left of the *kachel*. When I call your name, move to your right near the cubbies."

I glanced at the *kachel*; it was not lit. The room was icy.

"Hadassa and Sophie Wijzenbeek," the NSBer intoned after one of the officers said the self-same names. I wasn't sure why this needed interpretation.

With tears rolling unheeded down her cheeks, Zuster Deenik grabbed the flaxen-haired mischievous girl and her shy twin each by an arm and pulled them to where had been indicated.

"Georges and Elviere Baum."

Georges' green eyes cut left and right as if looking for an escape. There was none. With a deep sigh, he took his coughing five-year-old sister by the hand and trudged to join Hadassa and Sophie. Elviere sank to the floor. Seeing she wasn't healthy enough to remain standing, the Nazi officers left her there.

"Joseph and Bernard Waagenaar."

Tears filled my eyes as I remembered their tales of life at a farm in De Soetendael. A member of *het Verzet* (the Resistance) moved them to Driebergen. Evidently, that move wouldn't keep them safe.

Some children began to whimper, but the terrifying drone continued.

"Rosemarie Ida and Frieda Marianne van den Bergh."

Rosemarie carefully adjusted the bow in four-year-old Frieda's hair before putting an arm around her shoulder. Raising her chin, she walked toward where Zuster Deenik waited.

"Meriam, Edith, and Hans Wallig."

I felt my stomach clench as Meriam carried her 18-month-old baby brother to the other side of the room. Edith followed, tightly grasping her sister's skirt.

The crying escalated, and tears dripped from my chin.

"*Schweigen Allen!*" a blond officer with a skeletal face bit out before continuing in broken Dutch, "There's nothing to fear. We're just going to take these *kinderen* to their parents."

Zuster Dermout's face was carefully free of all emotion. Zuster Deenik seemed to have found something fascinating on the front of her apron, but I could see a sheen on her cheeks. That told me more than I wanted to know.

"Keet van Zanten."

My brown-eyed friend gave me a fearful glance before slowly making her way to the other side of the wall.

After a flurry of discussion, the officers continued, "Frits and Jan Evenblij."

I took my brother's hand before walking toward Keetie. There was no point resisting.

"*Nein* (no), not there. Come here. Stand in front of us."

Zuster Deenik gently pushed us toward the officers. Up close, I saw their eyes were the same color as a shark's. The expression was similar, too, and my knees knocked.

The soldiers leafed through their card file and had another heated discussion in German. I heard a few words I understood, like *Großvater* (grandfather), but none that unclenched my stomach.

"Pull down your shorts and underpants." The NSBer sounded bored.

I looked at Zuster Deenik. She nodded; her face was tight.

So, both Jan and I stood quaking with our pants around our ankles while the Nazis bent over the table to better observe our penises.

Whatever they saw appeared to help them make their decision. "They can go to the living room."

I quickly pulled up my pants before helping Jan with his.

Zuster Dermout opened the door. "Frits, Jan, you can leave."

"*De kinderen* whose names we didn't call can go, too," the NSBer droned.

Amongst the crush of terrified youngsters leaving the room, I glanced back at the children shivering by the fireplace. Would they let them go into the living room, too? Maybe after looking at their privates?

"Frits, stop your dreaming! Go!" Zuster Dermout's mouth was pinched, but her voice shook.

Pulling Jan closer, I turned away and followed Zuster Deenik, who was holding the door to the living room as if her life depended upon it.

After counting the children who were there, Zuster Deenik reached behind her to close the door. Just then, she stumbled forward, being hit by the very door that she was trying to shut. It flew open, and Keetie burst into the room, hair streaming behind her. She flung herself at me. "*Verstop me* (hide me), Fritsje, *verstop me!*"

"I...I...K...K...Keetie, Keetie,...how...where...what can I do?" My voice grew squeaky. I hugged her as I cast around for ideas but was powerless.

"Keet, you cannot be here." Zuster Deenik's fingers bit visibly into Keetie's upper arm. "Come with me. Hurry! Frits, you stay here."

All of us in the living room watched helplessly as the now-screaming Keetie was dragged from the room. I didn't notice the grief streaming down my cheeks until Jan reached over to touch my wet face. "Frits, why are you crying? Didn't you hear the officer? They're just going to their parents."

"Jean-Jean, I really, really hope that's t...t...true." I reluctantly joined the other children, who had their noses pressed to the window.

The Jewish children had been ushered out the back door and around the front, where they were loaded into the horse-drawn carriage usually used for our more special outings. One of the older children muttered that it looked like they would be going up the Traaij (the main street of Driebergen).

Just then, we saw Zuster Dermout running toward the cart as she struggled with her coat. "Please, Officers, let me go with them—at least as far as the train station!" Her sobs made it difficult to understand the words, but the smirking Nazi officers waited until she had climbed up with the children. As they left, I could hear the Jewish children, led by Zuster Dermout, singing a hymn.

"It's not fair!" pouted Trouble, "I bet they're going somewhere fun. I wish they'd chosen me to go."

"Be quiet and use your head if you can!" I exploded. "Remember Herman and Rosalie? Remember how our *Joodse kinderen* have always been kept hidden? It's daylight, and they're outside. Think!"

Once we'd been ushered back to the playroom, I sank to the floor with my head in my hands until Zuster Deenik and the kitchen help served us our meager supper of potatoes, endive, and gravy.

Afterward, I stumbled around the house collecting what trash there was. Sometimes, in the past, as I did the chores, I'd feel sorry for myself. Not now. I'd figured it out. Because our mother had elected not to have us circumcised, Jan and I weren't bound for the train station and the horrors that I was sure would come afterward.

That night, I found sleep more difficult to come by than it always was. Could I have helped Keetie and the other innocents? How could a mere boy protect another child? Surely, I could have figured out a hiding place! After all, I hadn't seen Jantje in the playroom. But where could I have hidden Keetie? And how? It had all happened so fast.

I turned over and gazed out of the window. Was Keetie looking at the same sky? What would happen to my cousins? How could I possibly explain to Mama that the enemy had taken her nieces and tiny nephew? Would the Nazis change their minds and come back for Jan and me once they reconsidered our heritage? How I wished Papa were still alive—he would have understood the ache in my heart without me needing to say a thing.

In the morning, the playroom was eerily quiet. The minuscule portion of buttermilk porridge we received tasted like sawdust. "Here, have mine, Jean-Jean," I whispered, surreptitiously exchanging my bowl for my brother's.

Just then, the rather red-eyed and pale-faced sisters came into the playroom. I'd heard that they and Jantje sometimes all shared a bed, so at least they had someone to cuddle during the night. But it was obvious that their sleep had been no better than mine.

Over two weeks later, there was news. "*Kinderen*," Zuster Dermout announced, "We're sorry to inform you that Hansje died."

Zuster Deenik wiped a tear from her cheek, but Zuster Dermout was stone-faced.

There was a collective gasp all around me, and I found it hard to breathe. Sweet, innocent, chubby little Hansje with his infectious grin, who'd just learned to toddle around on his fat legs, was dead. Dead! How could such a thing even be possible? He was so vibrantly alive. The darling of the children's home. I opened my mouth to ask for more information, but a look from Zuster Dermout stopped me.

A few months later, we had more bad news. Tante Bep had been crushed to death after having been enclosed in a nine square meter bunker with 74 other women at Kamp Vught. As if that weren't enough, some villagers told Zuster Dermout that Anni had been rounded up and presumably was also there. The warnings in the leaflets that the Germans constantly dropped and the talk around our village made me suspect we'd never see anyone who'd been taken ever again.

Knowing that those who hide Jews are severely punished, I wondered why Zusters Deenik and Dermout escaped a penalty but didn't ask. Could the nurses have been spared because of Burgemeester Tonnon and his friendship with Zuster Dermout's brother?

And how were our Jewish children discovered? I figured the nurses hadn't betrayed them since they cried when the Nazis took them away. Was it Meneer Flatow, who was now out of jail?

I felt terribly guilty because, despite having a Jewish grandparent, Jan and I remained free. Was it because Papa wasn't *Joods*? Didn't the Nazis know he was dead? After all, our cousins, who admittedly had a Jewish mother, had been taken. It all made no sense to me, especially because I knew that the children who were taken were both innocent and lovely. And I was not.

I remembered the hymn that first made such an impression while sitting next to Keetie. Could God help me "when darkness looms?" It seemed He had not helped her. He hadn't helped any of them.

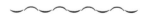

"Come Frits. Let's sit outside while Jan rides his bike. It's such a gorgeous day, but the weather won't last long. Sinterklaas is almost here."

I looked closely at Mama. Although she was, as usual, exquisitely turned out, her clothing was threadbare, and there were bags under her eyes. Her face was almost skeletal, and her hands trembled. It appeared that she, too, wasn't getting enough to eat. But I was certain more than that was wrong.

"What's going on, Mama? You look worried."

"I am. This war is lasting too long, and frankly, I wonder if any of us will survive."

"What do you mean? The soldiers haven't been back here since they took the *Joodse kinderen*."

"I know. The sisters keep us informed." Mama looked around and lowered her voice. "I've had more family news. Not long after picking up *de kinderen*, the Germans found Tante Esther and Oom Henri. They probably took them to Auschwitz, where I think your cousins are."

"Oh no! Have you heard? Are they okay?"

"I doubt it. She was pregnant yet again because the silly woman wanted to give your uncle a living son. She would have had the baby by now. But my NSB contact at work told me that Nazi physicians kill *Joodse* babies as soon as they're born. Stupid man thought I'd be impressed."

I covered my mouth. "They kill newborns—so my new cousin is dead, too?"

"Probably. The *Moffen* have no decency. Tante Esther is likely to be dead, too. They don't let the infirm remain alive." She shook her head. "Poor woman."

"What about Oom Henri?"

Mama shrugged. "I've heard nothing, so I'm going to keep believing *mijn broer* is as okay as he can be under the circumstances." She stood up, dusting off her coat. "Jan, let's go for a little walk. You can tell Mama how school has been going for you."

I stood, too. Dealing with pain by ignoring it still seemed to work for Mama. My eyes pricked with tears at the thought that my aunt and her baby were likely to be dead, but I decided to take a leaf out of her book. "I'd better go search for wood. Our stocks are getting low. If I'm not back by the time you go…bye, Mama."

Mama nodded, but her attention was already elsewhere, listening to my brother telling her just how much he hated school. I guessed she'd ignore that, as well.

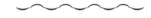

"Hey Jan, look! This fork is magic."

Jan dropped the picture book he was looking at to come and stand next to me, his eyes round. He was always game to see one of my tricks.

"Wow! That's amazing!" Trouble, who'd also drawn near, was almost as impressed as Jan. "How are you doing it?"

"I'm not. I t...t...told you. It's magic."

In almost no time, all the children in the playroom gathered around, watching the fork on the table move, seemingly of its own volition. I smirked. Sometimes, being the center of attention was fun.

Trouble bent and looked under the table. "Ha! A magnet! I caught you. But it was a cool trick."

I grinned. "I have another!" Taking a piece of beveled glass out of my pocket, I held it up to the light streaming through the window. "Look over there!"

All eyes followed to where I was pointing. A rainbow was dancing on the wall.

That trick could be improved upon. I manipulated the glass, and in no time, the rainbow was dancing on Zuster Deenik's behind. Not for long, since the ensuing giggles soon made her turn in our direction.

She glared at me, unsure of the source of our hilarity but suspecting that I'd been up to my usual tricks. "Frits, did you finish polishing the brass?"

"*Ja*, Zuster Deenik." Since the soldiers had confiscated most of it, that chore was easy.

"What about filling up the *kachel*?"

"*Ja*, Zuster Deenik."

"Are the windows clean?"

"*Ja*, Zuster Deenik." The sparkle in my eyes belied my poker face, but she was unable to see anything amiss, so shrugged and left the playroom.

As soon as the door closed, Trouble nudged me. "Can you do any other cool tricks?"

"*Ja*, watch this." Drawing a magnifying glass and a mirror out of my other pocket, I walked over to the window, where the sun was still high in the sky. I focused the light on the pages of a nearby book and reveled in the sounds of awe that resulted when a tiny curl of smoke began ascending to the ceiling.

"Umm, Frits, I think you'll get in big trouble if you set *het kindertehuis* on fire..." Trouble was frowning even as he bounced on his toes with eyes glued to the book.

Just then, the door opened again. I quickly slipped the mirror and glass into my pocket and closed the book, smothering the fire.

"What's that smell?" Zuster Dermout's long nose twitched just like a dog's.

I looked up innocently before exchanging glances with Trouble. Butter would not have melted in our mouths.

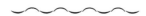

Juf van Kempen entered the playroom with red cheeks, her dress giving off the scent of fresh air. Schools had ceased operating, so she came to us instead. We immediately took our seats, waiting for the first lesson, but she slumped into a chair and just sat in silence. Trouble and I exchanged glances.

"Juffrouw? Are...are you okay?"

She inhaled deeply before expelling the breath. "Zuster Deenik just told me something so terrible. She heard it on...never mind. She heard it. Give me a minute."

"What?" I felt the onset of panic and squeezed my eyes shut as my breathing sped up.

"Putten." Juf van Kempen stopped for a few minutes before shaking her head. "I don't even know if I should tell you. Probably I shouldn't..."

"We hear gunfire every day; we've seen murders; tell us," Trouble observed with a twist in his mouth.

Eddie added, "Nothing will shock us."

"You're right. Sadly, by now, all of us are scarred for life. So, here it is. It's just so horrible—unimaginable. It happened in Putten, which is just north of us, you know."

"What? Just tell us!" My hands were again twirling.

"I am! Apparently, Nazi soldiers rounded up all the men and boys. They killed seven people outright, burned 100 homes, and deported over 650 men. The village now has almost no men left. Nobody knows why they did it, but it was probably another reprisal."

My mouth became like cotton as her words reminded me of what Jan and I saw not so long ago. Pictures of fathers thrown onto rose bushes and women crying formed in my mind. And the blood...so much blood.

I backed away from my beloved teacher, tempted to put my hands over my ears and scream at the top of my lungs, just like Jantje so often did.

Jan's whimper caught my attention.

"Oh, Jan, I didn't see you there. Are you okay, schatje (sweetheart)?" Juf van Kempen held out her arms.

Jan shook his head wordlessly, and I realized I needed to act quickly. I knew from experience that he'd react to human touch by crawling under a table and refusing to come out. "Jan, come here." I encircled him with my arm before explaining. "Juffrouw, Jan and I saw some reprisal shootings right here in Driebergen. It was just a few months ago. We didn't tell anyone, but it still upsets him."

"Oh, I'm so sorry. If I'd known…" She tucked her blond hair behind her ear with a trembling hand and muttered, "It's high time all of this was over."

After this incident, Juf van Kempen didn't come to *het kindertehuis* for several months. Trouble suggested that maybe she just found everything too stressful. Maybe she was scared. I imagined her hiding under a table and hoped that, with so many German soldiers leaving Driebergen, her absence was temporary. Maybe soon, Herr Hitler would have enough of fighting.

It was not to be. Instead, the churches and schools filled with refugees flooding east after their homes in Arnhem were bombed. The sight of ragged people with carts of household possessions tucked next to their wounded loved ones became commonplace. I heard rumors that Allied soldiers and Jews slept under the straw laid on the church floors while refugees slept on top, but had no idea how that would even work.

The Germans began raiding homes in Driebergen. They claimed they needed Dutch men to dig ditches and labor on railway lines. Few wanted to work for the enemy, but anyone who tried to escape or hide was shot. Soon, almost like Putten, there were no males left in our village. Well, except those who were either ancient or under 12 years old.

On Sunday, November 26, 1944, a deafening sound jolted me awake. We were used to gunfire and bombing, but this was different. The house shook, and Jan landed on my bed in a single leap. We wrapped our arms around each other, and I held my breath as I waited to die.

"*Kinderen*, come. To the cellar." Zuster Deenik stood at our bedroom door in her nightdress and cap. She raised her eyebrows at the fear-induced immobility of her charges. "Now! Quick!"

I jumped up, hurriedly gave Jan a sweater, and grabbed a couple of pairs of socks. We joined the silent line going down the stairs, along the hall, through the kitchen, through another door, and down a steep staircase with no railings. This dank place where potatoes were stored was nearly as frightening as the bombs. It had only one small window and a bare lightbulb. But the light was off, and it was still dark outside. I felt what I assumed was Jan's hand creep into mine and gripped it gratefully.

There we stood, the children, the two sisters, and the cook, just waiting. What had the Allies been aiming for? Would they bomb us, too?

After an hour of silence, Zuster Dermout told us it was safe to go upstairs and get dressed. Then we would have what breakfast there was. We later heard that most of the damage had been in Doorn, where the Allies destroyed some German warplanes hidden in the forest.

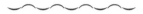

My restless shifting around on the cold, hard pew earned me a warning frown, so I fell to picking my hangnails. The pastor was talking, but I wasn't particularly interested in what he had to say. The intricacies of nature and the wonder of my now-deceased baby cousin convinced me there is a creator, and he, she, or it must be brilliant. But what we'd seen during the war surely proved that the creator didn't care about, much less love, us. We'd been forgotten.

Just then, the pastor said something so utterly unreasonable that my body became as still as a stone. All except my rather oversized ears. They swiveled in his direction. "The Bible tells us we will only be forgiven if we forgive."

I sucked in my lips. Surely, he was lying! Closing my eyes, I recalled the Lord's prayer, which we'd all been forced to memorize. "…Forgive us our sins as we forgive those who sin against us…" Hmm, maybe he was right—it did say that.

I thought back to the Nazi soldiers who I'd seen kill two men. How could their families and the woman they raped ever forgive them? What about the bombing of Doorn? Sure, the Allies were on our side, but innocent civilians had died. Would the grieving loved ones forgive? Should they? I didn't even want to think about my dead friends and relatives.

And, although I might have earned some of the blows dealt by Zuster Dermout, I was sure I didn't deserve them all. What was worse was that my pain was devastating to Jan. How could I forgive her? Why would I want to?

The pastor continued. "With everything happening in our country, you may wonder why God would demand something that seems so unreasonable. Of course, we know Jesus forgave His enemies from the cross, and we're told to follow His example. But He's God, and we're only human."

I nodded my head and crossed my arms. The command to forgive was utterly ridiculous and unfair. My childish misdemeanors were hardly comparable to murder.

"So, why would God require something like this? It's because He loves us. It's not for the benefit of our enemies; they may never even know we forgave them. It's for our own sake. You see, hanging on to wrath harms the person who's angry far more than it does the person they're mad at. God doesn't want us to suffer more."

I glanced at Trouble to see what he thought about what was being said. He was gazing at the stained-glass windows and picking his nose. No help there.

Closing my eyes, I saw Keetie's hands flying over the piano keys and the fear in her face as she was taken away. I remembered Meriam's laughing eyes as we shared a joke and her trembling voice as we shared confidences in the stairwell. I heard Hansje's giggle as I chased him around the playroom and saw his innocent hand gripping Meriam's shoulder. The pastor obviously didn't know that some things are unforgivable. So, forgiveness? Nope. Not going to happen. Not going to forgive. Even if God does exist.

I dismissed what the pastor said. But I remembered it.

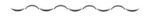

Trouble's nose wrinkled as he pushed the mess on his plate from side to side. "Yum," he drawled under his breath. "Potato peels and chickweed."

"I think I see a piece of mushroom there. I found a couple in the *het bos*." I forked a disgusting bite into my mouth and closed my eyes. "Mmm, delicious! Eat and be grateful!"

Jan sighed and whispered. "This makes yesterday's offal and berries seem like gourmet food."

"Silence!" Hunger had not sweetened Zuster Dermout's disposition at all.

The simple fact was that there was very little food to be bought. The central shopping street of Driebergen resembled a ghost town. Shops formerly owned by Jews were abandoned, their windows broken. Shelves in stores that were still open were mostly empty.

I was proud to discover a shop that still had rope. The sisters bought some to hold up our pants, a great help when skinny kids are playing tag or doing semi-naked exercises in the garden.

Unless I was searching for firewood, visits to the forest were no longer permitted. No more catching newts and climbing trees. The Nazis had taken our bikes, not that we had the energy to ride. Our outdoor entertainment consisted of standing in the backyard, watching dogfights, and talking.

With his eyes glued to the sky, Eddie asked, "Why do you think the *vieze rot Moffen* need our school building?"

"Who knows?" Appie shrugged. "They can't sit there. All the desks were burned for fuel a long time ago."

"Haven't you seen the lines of people walking to and from school? They're keeping *Joden* there until it's their turn to go to the train station." Hans's eyes were narrowed.

"Where Juf van Kempen said they're shipped to their deaths," Trouble whispered.

My shoulders rounded. This too was absolutely unforgivable.

Although our teacher sometimes came to *het kindertehuis*, her visits were less frequent than they had been. Her favorite subjects seemed to be the writings of Aristotle, Plato, and Aquinas; her ultimate goal was to encourage us to think. She was taking a colossal risk in what she was teaching, let alone coming at all. I loved her all the more because of it; she gave me some of what Mama didn't.

By now, I thought I was used to the continual blows life dealt me. I walked in a fog; nothing touched me. Or so I thought. Strangely, Mama's next visit was the final straw.

Papa's last letter to Frits—just four days before he passed.

den Haag, 22 Juli 1942.

Lieve Frits,

Zoo, mijn jongen, ben je over-
gegaan. Wat fijn, hé, Papa is
er ook erg blij om en Mama zal
het ook zijn als ik het haar
vertel. Mama is een paar dagen
naar Amsterdam met vacantie,
als zij terugkomt zal ik graag
jouw brief laten lezen, hoor.
Ik vind dat je mooie cijfers
hebt. Wanneer krijgen jullie
vacantie of heb je het mis-
schien al? Het weer is niet zoo
mooi nu, veel te koud en te
regenachtig om te gaan zwemmen.
Je schiet al aardig op met
de zwemles, hé Frits. Als je naar

Papa toekomt zal je dan het
diploma meebrengen om te laten
zien. Met Papa gaat het weer
niet zoo goed, ik verlang heel
erg naar mijn groote zoon en
naar broertje.
Dag lieve jongens, veel
liefs en een heeleboel
zoentjes van pappa

120

School photo in Driebergen. Frits is at the far left; Juf van Kempen is at the back on the left; Jantje is in the middle at the back, and CW Siegers is at the back on the right, 1943. (top)

Frits takes Jan to school on his bicycle, 1942. (bottom)

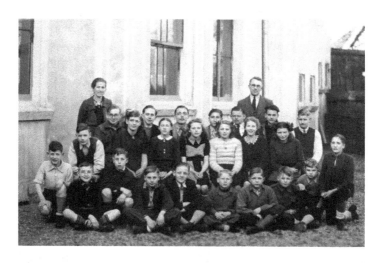

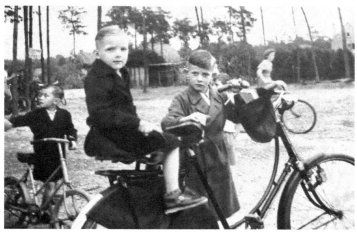

Frits and Jan in the snow in Driebergen, 1942. (top)

Newborn Hansje Wallig, 1942. (bottom)

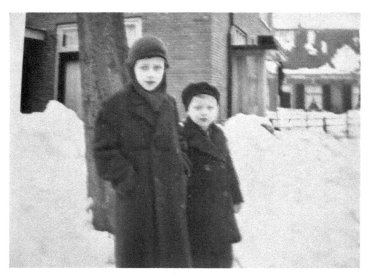

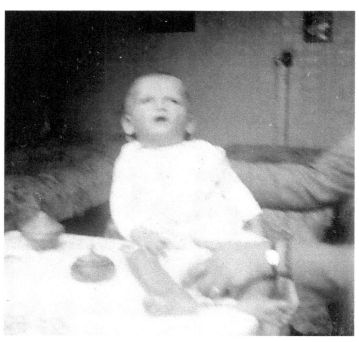

7

THE INFIRMITY

"Frits and Jan, your mother is here to see you."

I sighed and put away the crossword I'd been working on. Mama had been coming more frequently since she'd found a job and a room nearby, but I didn't care. Her visits were always a test of my endurance.

Zuster Deenik indicated that we should go to the living room, where more official social calls were sometimes conducted. Mystified, I opened the door, stopped short, and pushed Jan behind me. A tall, extremely handsome, dark-haired man sat on the couch beside Mama. Who was he? And why were the curtains drawn, even though it was daytime? The hair on the back of my neck stood to attention.

"Come in, boys. I have someone I'd like you to meet. This is Meneer Eduard Goudsmit."

I pressed my lips together. Why was she introducing us to this man, who even to my young eyes appeared to be Jewish? Why bring him to *het kindertehuis*, which was clearly a risk to him, if not to all of us?

Mama's eyes were bright, and her cheeks were flushed. "Meneer Goudsmit and I are engaged. We'll be married as soon as the war is over. Then, he'll be your new father."

I narrowed my eyes and pressed my lips together, but Mama ignored the warning in my face.

"Frits and Jan, don't just stand there. Come and shake his hand."

Jan, devoid of expression, approached and stuck out his hand. I put mine behind my back.

"Frits!" Mama warned before turning to her fiancé. "I told you he's difficult."

The man chuckled and started to reply, but I interrupted.

"*Nee,* I'm not! I'm angry—very angry!" My eyes were blazing, and if they could have shot bullets, Mama would have been dead. "Papa is still my father, and I don't need anyone else." Heedless of her embarrassed protests, I turned on my heel and left the room.

My young shadow followed and stood beside me as I faced the hallway wall with clenched fists. "It's not her fault Papa died, you know," Jan whispered. "Your life would be easier if you just let things happen."

I ground out, "I'm not you," between clenched teeth.

The following day, I awoke with crushing pain in my chest. Barely able to draw a breath, I banged my hand on the headboard to wake someone, anyone, up.

"What?" Trouble's sleepy voice asked.

"Get...Sister...help!" was all I could manage.

My friend leaped out of bed to peer at me. Then he ran. The sisters wouldn't be happy with a child invading their bedroom, but this was an emergency.

Next thing I knew, Zuster Deenik, her hair in a scarf, was standing at my bedside. "What's the problem?"

"Hurts!" I gasped, rubbing my chest. "So much!"

The sister grabbed my wrist, took out her pocket watch, and began counting. Her face grew pale. "Dirk, run and wake Zuster Dermout up. Tell her to get Dokter Hermans right away. RUN!"

By now, the room was swimming, and I was gasping for breath.

Zuster Deenik grasped my shoulders and gave me a little shake. "Frits, listen to me! You're fine—it's just a bit of pain from eating too fast."

My eyes met hers. Although Zuster Deenik's urgent tones belied her words, she had my attention.

"Okay now. Do as I say. It'll make the pain recede. Imagine you're lying down in a peaceful meadow, and the sun is on your face. Watch the clouds floating by in the blue sky. The birds are singing. The flowers smell wonderful."

As I listened to her gravelly voice painting a beautiful picture, I felt Jan's hand slip into mine. My breath slowed, and the tightness in my chest eased. Zuster Deenik gently tucked the covers around me.

I was just drifting off to sleep, dreaming that my feet were immersed in a babbling brook, when I became aware of whispers. The person holding my wrist was now Dr. Hermans, and he was talking with both sisters. Standing behind them, their faces screwed up with worry, were Trouble and Jan.

"Oh, you're awake. I'm just going to listen to your heart, okay?"

I silently pushed the blanket down and lifted my pajama top.

The stethoscope was icy in the cold room, but it was the resurgence of crushing pain that made me catch my breath. Zuster Deenik resumed her gentle monologue while stroking my hair, encouraging me to relax through the pain.

Dr. Hermans pursed his lips and then ran his hands over my knees and elbows. Once he'd finished his exam, he stepped away from my bed. The doctor spoke in a whisper, but I had young ears. "I'm hearing some worrying sounds—his heart is not doing well. It's going far too fast."

"Oh, dear! We've had so much sickness," Zuster Dermout lamented. "Coughs. Sore throats. Scarlet fever. He had such a bad time with that one. I so much hoped his health would improve by now."

"Scarlet fever? I didn't know that'd been through here, too. This all makes sense now. In some children, that illness can progress to rheumatic fever, which damages the heart. Has he been complaining that his elbows and knees hurt?"

Zuster Deenik shrugged and shook her head. "They all complain when we have them exercise in the morning. Especially about moving the stick around their heads. It's hard to know whose complaint is genuine."

"His were. Come here." Dr. Hermans guided Zuster Deenik's hand. "Can you feel these nodules under his skin? That's a bad sign."

"Oh, dear! Will he be okay? What can we do?" Zuster Deenik's hands shook as she tucked the covers around me once again.

"Keep him warm, preferably inside and away from drafts. No strenuous exercise for at least three months. He should only sit in a chair or lie on a bed. And he should be calm; shocks and worrying could kill him. His heart and body both need time to heal—and even then they may not. Maybe see if the butcher can provide you with a bone to make broth for him."

So it was that I spent months engaged in not much of anything except playing chess, reading, and doing puzzles. The sisters did their best to keep me from stress, but they could do little about the memories that stubbornly refused to remain where they'd been stuffed. Assistance with those came from my beloved teacher, Juf van Kempen, who spent hours near her troubled pupil, just listening to the waterfall of his grief.

Sitting near the *kachel* while we gathered at her feet, Juf van Kempen shared what she'd heard on Radio Oranje. "*Kinderen*, there's both good news and bad news. The good is that the Allies are on their way to Germany. They've liberated much of our country, mostly the regions south of us. The bad news is they've bypassed us since we're not of strategic importance. We're successfully sabotaging railways and telephone lines to help the Allies, but our occupation isn't over yet."

Hans jumped to his feet. "Will we be free soon?"

"Oh, I should think so. The Germans are running out of soldiers, and the Allies are making so much progress. We'll soon experience some relief from this war."

Juf van Kempen was wrong in her predictions, as were many others. The Germans retaliated against the railway strike by not allowing food to reach our part of the country. By the time they lifted the embargo, fearing the chaos that could result, it was too late. Those farmers who had been sending us what little food they produced had switched to supplying the black market. Bridges, docks, and roads had been destroyed so nothing could get through. The winter was harsh, and the canals froze. There was no gas and electricity and no food. It was the Hunger Winter.

Since my heart trouble began, Jan had been doing my chores. But I was slowly feeling stronger, and with improved health came guilt. I'd promised my father to take care of my brother, not vice versa. He was coughing incessantly, and I feared tuberculosis. "Jan, it's freezing outside. How about you do the inside jobs, like polishing the brass, peeling potatoes, and cleaning the shoes? I'll collect firewood, chop logs, fill the *kachel*, and take out the garbage."

Jan wrinkled his nose. "I hate doing the shoes. The other kids see me. They laugh at me."

"Okay, I'll do the shoes if you do the garbage. But you have to wear two sweaters when you do it and lend me your sweater when I'm outside." Secretly, I was relieved. Taking out the garbage really bothered me—with no soap, no amount of hand washing could get rid of the stench. I'd do anything to be rid of that chore.

"Deal!"

I glanced out of the window at the nonexistent wood pile and sighed. "Hand it over." Layering the two sweaters with my threadbare coat and packing my shoes with scraps of paper, I trudged out into the snow, once again pulling the creaky wagon.

"Hey, Frits, want company?"

"*Ja, bedankt*! Nothing like a bit of Trouble to help me collect wood."

I received the punch on my arm in the spirit he offered it. "So, where should we go?"

"I think by the monastery. The soldiers living there won't be out in this weather. And, since everyone else is scared to go near them, we might find more wood."

Bent double against the wind, Trouble and I walked down the street until we were near our goal.

"Let's go this way." I tugged Trouble's arm toward a path into the woods, and we began our search for sticks. Suddenly, I felt a splat against my hat, and cold snow made its way down my neck and back.

"I can't believe you did that!" I shouted, chasing after Trouble. He scampered away, laughing hysterically.

I bent, scooped up a handful of snow, and launched my missile. I missed. Trouble, that is.

"Hey!" The enraged voice almost made me wet my pants. Being focused on our game, I hadn't noticed the German soldier. Now I could see the imprint of my snowball on his chest!

His mouth was a tight white knot, and his narrowed eyes threw daggers at me before he turned toward where Trouble was hiding. "You there, I see you, so you might as well come out."

Trouble sheepishly emerged from the trees. "He was aiming at me, *Herr Soldat*." His voice trembled.

With raised eyebrows, the soldier smirked before he observed, "But he hit me."

"I'm sorry." I hung my head and hoped for mercy while trying to rub the pain in my chest away.

The German stroked the gun hung over his shoulder; I prepared to die. I could hear the woman crying after the men were shot and looked around for rose bushes. After a few tense minutes, he spoke. "There's something you can do for me."

I looked up in surprise. Maybe I'd survive until tomorrow. Well, if my racing heart didn't give out.

"Get me tobacco for cigarettes." He held out some money.

My heart sank. "Sir, they don't have any. The store ran out a long time ago."

Trouble nodded his head vigorously, corroborating my story.

"Boy, I want cigarettes. Don't make me angrier than I already am. Go get me some." He thrust the coins into my hand.

I backed away, clutching the guilders. "Okay, I'll go, and if they have tobacco, I'll bring it. I promise."

"Me, too." Trouble was only too anxious not to be left behind.

We left the wagon where it was and ran to the tobacconist, bursting through the door. "We need tobacco!"

"Too bad. We don't have any. Haven't had any for over a year. Anything else?" The shopkeeper inspected his nails and whistled tunelessly.

"Now what?" whispered Trouble.

I opened the door. "Umm, we need to go back and tell him."

"Not a chance! I'm out of here!"

I watched my unfaithful friend's quickly disappearing form before plodding back to face the soldier. He was bound to be furious. I felt sick to my stomach but tried to reason philosophically: it'd be better if only one of us died, anyway.

"Sir, they don't have any tobacco. Here's your money."

The soldier, who'd been lounging against the building with his ankles crossed, stood straight to peer behind me.

"Where's your friend?"

I pulled a face and shrugged. "He's not coming. He was too scared."

"Is that so? Well then, you're lucky."

"Why?" By now, I was shivering from both cold and fear.

"I only shoot cowards. Keep the money." The soldier turned away and walked into the monastery, leaving me with my mouth open. I ran back to *het kindertehuis* as fast as my legs could carry me. Just in case he changed his mind.

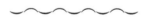

1945 "You look like a skeleton! Your eyes are sunken into their sockets, and I can count your ribs." Trouble stood with his hands on his hips, unashamedly examining me while I washed my face in cold water.

I sent a splash in his direction. "Have you looked at your own knobbly knees? And look at your fat belly. Maybe you're a girl because it sure looks like you're expecting a baby!"

"Ha! I'm not a girl. You're a girl!"

It was February, but the cold weather showed little sign of abating, and with the stricter curfews, foraging for wood wasn't advisable. Food had become scarce, even for us outside the big cities.

The pain that goes with hunger was my constant companion, and I wondered if I would survive the war, not that I cared.

We all knew not to complain of stomach aches since the sisters would force us to drink six large glasses of warm water as a "cure." When we vomited, they would declare us better. The result? None of us dared to say anything.

It was, however, impossible to suppress sickness in this manner. By now, retching, groans, and coughing were commonplace in *het kindertehuis*. More and more children succumbed to dysentery and tuberculosis. The kitchen staff, with little but sugar beets to cook, helped with clean-up and nursing, but there was still too much for the adults to cover. After all, they also had very little food and heat.

I lay on Jan's bunk in our icy bedroom, my body curled around his. We huddled under both our blankets. He had just turned nine but was the size of someone much younger. "Frits, I'm so cold! Can you get me another blanket?" My brother's cheeks were rosy, and his teeth were chattering. He was putting off enough heat to warm a room.

I shook my head as I pushed his hair off his forehead. "Zuster Deenik said we don't have extra. I'll hold you closer until your fever breaks. Then, you'll feel better."

"Will my tummy stop hurting, too?"

"Yeah, I think so. Surely, that last poop got rid of all the sickness."

Just then, the door opened. "How's he doing?" Zuster Dermout's voice was almost bearable as she lowered it so as not to disturb the sick.

"Not well. He can't keep anything down—not even water."

"Oh dear. Just keep offering him a spoon of water once in a while. Hopefully, he'll soon turn the corner." Zuster Dermout bent over to do what was usually my job. She set down a clean bucket, exchanging it for the one that was full of vomit and bloody diarrhea.

Trouble popped his head around the door. "Zuster Dermout, it's Jantje. Zuster Deenik says to come quickly. I'll go get Dr. Hermans."

Zuster Dermout's emaciated face grew even more pale, and she set the stinking bucket down. She then ran to the room the sisters shared with the now 15-year-old Jantje. I was reminded of the whispered speculation about the young man: he was clearly a favorite. Could he be an illegitimate son? Or was he favored (and hidden) because of his disability, which by Nazi rules should have landed him in the camps?

A hush fell over *het kindertehuis* when the doctor came down, followed by the sisters, who both had tear-filled eyes. Trouble was the one who told me that Jantje was seriously ill. They didn't even know if he would survive.

I immediately returned to our room and held my sleeping brother tightly. "Fight Jean-Jean! Get better for me." I didn't leave my brother's side for the next two days and nights except to get him more water. And then, slowly, he recovered. Jantje, who had Zuster Deenik's undivided attention, did too.

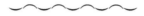

Zuster Deenik called Jan and me in from the garden area, where we were sitting on the grass, having no energy for activity. "Your mother's here, boys. Wash up and go in."

Before entering the living room, I carefully straightened Jan and my clothing and hair. Mama didn't like her sons to look untidy.

"Mama." My brother mirrored Mama as he greeted her without emotion while I stood in shock. Mama hadn't visited since the start of the Hunger Winter, but that wasn't the reason for my surprise.

Although we were all emaciated by now, Mama looked worse than terrible. Her eyes were red, her hair dull, and she was slumped in the chair. She whose back was usually ramrod straight. Even her clothing was rumpled.

"Mama? Are you sick?"

Our mother shook herself and attempted a bright smile, but it looked more like a grimace. "I'm fine…well, not really." She passed her hand over her face. "Oh, this is impossible!"

I bit my lip. Mama seemed far more upset than she was when Papa died or even when she related that our aunt and baby had been murdered. What could be wrong? Was she dying? Had someone else died? But who was left? I swallowed hard.

My mother took a deep breath and continued. "I might as well tell you. When the Allies bombed the Bezuidenhout, they hit the apartment where our family possessions were. All the lovely furniture, pictures, and carvings from the Congo burned up."

I frowned before asking about what I considered the most important thing. "Do you have any photos of Papa left?"

"A couple. And a few of you as babies. But not many." Mama shrugged before continuing. "And, as if that were not enough, well..." She took a deep breath. "You remember Meneer Goudsmit? You met him. I was so lonely after your father passed…"

Jan snorted. "And we, being left here, aren't?"

Mama ignored his outburst and continued. "Well...he's dead, too. He was arrested after *het Verzet*'s failed assassination attempt on General Hanns Rauter. The Nazis kept him in prison for some time, but he was executed a couple of days ago."

She dashed away a tear, but Jan shrugged. "Huh, didn't know he was part of *het Verzet*."

I opened my mouth to comment on the known risks, then closed it again. Obviously, she knew. And what could I say? The idea that she'd moved on from Papa when I still had a gaping hole in my heart infuriated me, so it was better to remain silent.

I knew something of grief and sorrow after losing Keetie and wouldn't wish it on anyone, but this was my mother. I doubted she was even capable of feeling. However, perhaps if the sorrow was her own... In the end, I ignored the elephant in the room.

I shrugged. "Well, I'm sorry for your losses. But let me tell you about the chess championship I won here in *het kindertehuis*. I beat Appie!"

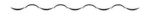

"What's that sound?" Trouble asked.

With the coming of Spring, the sisters occasionally allowed those of us who weren't too ill to spend time outside.

I stood still to listen. "I'm not sure. It sounds like someone sawing wood, but it's not coming from the direction of *het bos*."

Trouble glanced over his shoulder to be sure the nurses weren't watching. "Let's go see!"

"Can I come?"

"Of course, Jan. That is if you can keep up..."

Following the sound, we turned from the Traaij onto the Hoofdstraat. Curiosity won out over starvation-induced lethargy.

Our eyes widened upon seeing German soldiers carving notches in the trunks of all the trees lining the street. We drew closer, being careful to stay out of sight. Other soldiers were following them, stuffing something into the notches. What were they doing?

Suddenly, *boom!* We three boys jumped and clutched each other. My heart was pounding so loud that I was sure it was audible.

"What was that?" I mouthed.

Trouble pointed silently. A tree was lying across the road at the end of the street, where they'd evidently begun their sawing.

We continued to watch. One by one, there was an explosion, and each tree fell across the road. When the soldiers drew near to our hiding place, we returned to the garden of *het kindertehuis*.

"Why do you think they're doing that?" Trouble cocked his head on one side.

"Who knows why the *vieze rot Moffen* do anything, but one thing is for sure. Nobody is going to be driving down that street."

Jan giggled at my words—he knew filthy language was definitely forbidden. I made a mental note to use it more often. I missed that sound, and who knew how much longer any of us would even be around?

8

THE LIBERATION

My 12th birthday came and went virtually without recognition, but it brought the best gift of all. Just two days afterward, on May 5, Juf van Kempen burst into the playroom, her hollow cheeks red and her eyes shining. "Come outside, everybody. Come see!"

Zuster Dermout frowned. "See what?"

"We've been liberated! Surely, the end of the war is near—and for us, it's now."

The room had been quiet, but no more. We filed out of the garden and gleefully joined the virtual stampede of people walking up the Traaij to the Hoofdstraat. Allied soldiers drove their tanks right over the fallen trees as we and the village people shouted, "*Het is vrede! Het is vrede* (It is peace)!"

"Now we know why they did it," I snickered. "Didn't work."

"It'll all be better now." Trouble paused in thought and then sighed. "Maybe we'll finally get more food and be able to have heat. Or even leave our yard after dark…"

We were disappointed. The German soldiers didn't leave quietly. Instead, they became more vindictive, shooting people on sight for no reason other than that they were there.

The shops weren't suddenly filled with food. Bridges and railways needed to be rebuilt; decimated farms had to begin once again functioning—an almost impossible task when so many men were missing. The Red Cross dropped care packages over big cities, but we were just a town. Nothing came to us.

Our friends, relatives, and acquaintances were still dead. With the absence of daily fear came a resurgence of grief. I later learned the fates of the children taken from *het kindertehuis*. Some, including Keetie, went via Weteringschans to the orphanage at Westerbork. After only three weeks, they were transported to Auschwitz, where they were murdered, presumably in the gas chambers. Well, all except Hadassa and Sophie. As twins, they first underwent two days of torturous medical experiments. The rest of the children, my cousins included, were transported to Auschwitz on February 8 and died three days later. Every one of them. My aunt and eight of the children taken from Welgelegenlaan were killed on the same day. Seventy-five percent of our Jewish population was dead. Unforgivable.

On Monday, May 7, 1945, Germany surrendered unconditionally, even though the end of the war overseas would take until September.

Mama came to see us a couple of months later.

"Mama, did you hear? The war is over. We're free!" Jan was still pale from recent starvation, but his eyes shone.

"*Ja*, Zuster Deenik phoned and told me when it happened. Finally, life can return to normal."

"We can come home now, right?" Jan asked while I pondered her words. How could life ever be normal without Papa, Tante Esther, our cousins, and Keetie?

Mama shook her head and forced a laugh. "*Nee*, Jan, whatever gave you that idea? I'm still a widow and need to earn money to live. I can't take care of both of you, as well. My life will remain hard."

I grimaced while rubbing my chest. "Will *het k...k...kindertehuis* remain open since all the *Joodse kinderen* are gone and the war is over? The sisters seem exhausted. I think they may want a break."

"Nonsense! Everyone has suffered, but now we all need to pull together." A shadow passed over Mama's face. "Even me."

There was a moment of silence while I wondered at the extreme sadness on her face. Had something more happened, something of which I'd been unaware? I decided I didn't care, but I did have another question.

"Mama, Radio Oranje said the Russians liberated Auschwitz way back in January. Have you heard from Oom Henri? Did he survive?"

"I did hear. He's been free for a month or so and is living with Tante Aleida. Of course, his possessions were destroyed when my house was bombed."

"But Auschwitz was liberated a long time ago!"

"He wasn't there when it was liberated. Being one of the few men strong enough to survive, Oom Henri first had to walk to another camp. That's where the Canadians found him."

"Can we see him when we next go to Scheveningen?"

"*Nee*, absolutely not. He's still very sick and weak." Mama took a deep breath. "I think maybe he's lost his mind. I never want to hear about him again." Her sharp nod and pursed lips meant the subject was permanently closed.

Jan opened his mouth, and I nudged him. There was definitely a story here. However, it was obvious we wouldn't get more out of Mama. Oom Henri definitely suffered enough for him to lose his sanity: he'd lost his wife and four children, his home, and his health. None of it was his fault! So why in the world was Mama so furious with him?

That night, I mulled over the questions that were still fighting for my attention. Why did Nazi officers decide to let us live but not our cousins? Was it truly just our penises? Why was our uncle taken to Auschwitz but not Mama, who didn't even bother to hide? Why didn't the Nazis punish Zusters Dermout and Deenik, who'd been hiding Jewish children? Why didn't they take Jantje, who was just what the Nazis hated: disabled? Who betrayed us?

I punched my pillow, remembering that whenever I asked Juf van Kempen any of my questions, she quickly changed the subject. It was unlikely I'd ever find the answers. Truthfully, I wasn't even sure I wanted to. I was just so angry, and I wasn't alone.

Since liberation, irate Dutch people attacked anyone suspected of collaborating with the enemy. On one of our wood-gathering trips, Jan and I witnessed a gang of men shaving the heads of young women. The girls had been too friendly with German soldiers. Later, we saw some town youngsters following those same women with a long stick. They were removing the scarves with which the girls hid their shame, doubtless thinking it was great sport. My fists clenched. I'd seen enough cruelty, and this harassment infuriated me.

The sisters were also enraged and decided to take vengeance on Meneer Flatow. Trouble and I overheard them speaking with Detectives Van Pelt and Van der Linden of the Rotterdam Political Investigation Service. The detectives advised the sisters to write a letter to accuse S. Werner Flatow of betraying our Jewish children, and they did. They believed he used them as a bargaining chip in his efforts to have his smuggling sentence reduced. It seemed to have worked. He went free while Anni Amalie was murdered. The court eventually decided not to prosecute him, but in my opinion, something was fishy.

Some of the NSBers, including Burgemeester Tonnon, were arrested and imprisoned, but not all. After all, three percent of our men were active in the party that had helped the Germans. With so many dead, it wasn't feasible to lock up the guilty survivors—but I wished we could.

Honestly, I was seething with anger—at Mama, at Flatow, at Tonnon, at the NSBers, at the entire German nation, but firmly buried my head in the sand. That made breathing difficult, but at least it kept my rage from exploding.

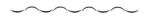

I came out of the water sputtering, spotted Trouble, and jumped on his head, pushing him under. With the very gradual increase in food, our energy was returning, as was our tendency toward getting into deep water—sometimes literally.

"Frits! Dirk! None of that! Swim five laps."

We grinned at each other. This was not as much of a punishment as Zuster Deenik imagined. We frequently joked that we were half boy and half fish.

Our laps completed, Dirk came over to me with bulging cheeks. A warm spray of water hit me in the face. I gave him a shove.

"I can't believe you did that, you *lul* (penis)."

"Well, you're the *stommert* (dumb guy) who got in my way."

"Dirk, I heard that. Get out of the pool." Busted!

Smirking, I nonchalantly swam a few laps of backstroke, waving at my friend each time I passed. But only when Zuster Deenik was looking elsewhere.

After two hours of fun, the sisters ordered all the children to get out, dress, and return to *het kindertehuis.*

Once dry, I grabbed my bike, and Jan rode up to join me.

"Hey, Frits, let's go back via the Traaij. I saw an amazing cup in a window there. I want to show it to you."

"Um, that's not exactly on the way back."

"Yeah, but if we go fast, they'll never know."

A cup was not incredibly high on my list of marvels, but my withdrawn brother had no friends. He needed someone to pay attention to him.

I gave a quick nod. "I'll race you!" We completed the journey in record time.

"Look!" Jan hopped off and pointed to a cup decorated with a Dutch flag, an apple, an orange, and a portrait of the queen. It really was singularly ugly.

I forced what I hoped was an impressed smile. "Wow! That's…really…something!"

Jan sighed and spoke dreamily. "It's so beautiful. I wish I could buy it."

There was little I could say, so I decided a subject change was in order. "Well, let me show you something else. Remember how mean the shopkeeper in this store was when we asked if we could buy some *zuurtjes*?"

"Umm, *ja*?"

"Well, watch this."

The shopkeeper wasn't behind the counter, so I pulled a magnifying glass out of my pocket and focused it on some paper in the window.

"What are you doing?" Jan whispered, even while keeping his eyes glued to the paper.

"I'm gonna set the shop on fire. He deserves it."

Jan held his breath, anticipating that glorious moment when things would burst into flames. Then he grabbed my arm.

"Frits! Stop!"

I shook myself free. "Be patient, Jan. I've nearly got it."

"*Nee,* Frits. Stop!" Jan sounded like he was hyperventilating— or about to pee his pants. Just as I was turning to see what was the matter, I heard a familiar strident voice. The hair on the back of my neck stood on end.

"Frits, come with me."

My precious magnifying glass disappeared into the abyss of Zuster Dermout's pocket, and I spent the rest of the day locked in the attic. No food. No drink. No light. Only the memory of those who hid here. All so I would learn my lesson.

I didn't. Instead, I spent the time figuring out where I could procure another magnifying glass.

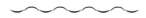

"It's almost Sinterklaas. Do you think we'll get anything from Mama?"

I shook my head. "Jan, the shop windows are still empty. And, really, we're too old for all that nonsense."

"Yeah, I guess you're right." Jan's rounded shoulders told me nine years old wasn't too old.

My brow furrowed as I tried to figure out how to make Sinterklaas memorable for my brother. Could I get money? Was there something else I could trade for candy or even a present? Could I make something Jan would enjoy?

As the day approached, I grew more desperate. Having worked through their anger, the entire country was engaged in over-the-top Sinterklaas celebrations, doubtless fueled by collective relief. But I still didn't have any money.

Trouble tapped his nose and winked. "I know what you could do. Offer to make a couple of deliveries for the shopkeeper in exchange for *zuurtjes*."

"Will you cover for me?"

"Sure! I'll say you're out searching for wood. But be sure to bring some back when you return."

Unfortunately, this plan required cooperation from the shopkeeper. I got wood, but no candy.

On the morning of Sinterklaas, I prepared myself mentally to console my brother. Therefore, my eyes bugged out as the nurses came in carrying huge bags of candy. My mouth (and eyes) watered as they poured it out in front of the smaller children. Jan got his candy after all, and I refused to accept his offer of even one piece.

With sticky fingers and chocolate-smeared faces, the children were then herded onto a makeshift stage where they performed a show for us older children. It went as well as could be expected.

In the afternoon, we older children got our treat. We were going to go to Driebergen's free theater while the very young children rested. The great thing was that, while Jan was considered young in terms of getting candy, he was old enough to go to the theater. Double dipping!

"Hurry, *kinderen!*" Zuster Deenik's flushed cheeks made me grin. She looked as excited as her charges.

"What'll we see?" Trouble asked.

"More than you'd believe! First, a magician will perform, and then there'll be two miniplays."

Jan's eyes grew round. So much entertainment in just one afternoon! He led the way out the door and up the street to the theater.

"Hey, Trouble, sit here beside me," I invited. "Jan is on my other side."

We sat on the edge of our seats, waiting until the curtain rose. First up was the magician. I watched him closely to see if I could figure out how he did his tricks. Some were obvious, but I had no idea how he got that rabbit out of his hat.

Doktor Know-all was pretty funny and seriously tickled Jan's funny bone. His giggles were what made me grin. But the highlight of my afternoon was the portrayal of Abu Kassim, a story from the *Thousand and One Nights*. I laughed until my stomach hurt seeing the old Egyptian miser trying to rid himself of the smelly shoes he stole— again and again.

By the time we returned to *het kindertehuis*, Zuster Dermout had given up on getting the highly-sugared children to nap. We ate an early dinner; the table was cleared, and we were instructed to sit on the floor.

When the expected knock at the door came, I wasn't worried. I knew Piet didn't know if I'd been bad or good, so strode forward confidently when summoned by the sisters. What made me stagger was the number of gifts I received. Six! A huge diary, a pencil case, pencils, a tie, an educational game, a cardboard building plate, and lots of candy! No magnifying glass, but that wasn't surprising. Mama probably heard what I tried to do with the last one.

To complete a fantastic day, the older children were allowed to stay up playing games until 11:00. Even Jan.

Christmas isn't celebrated with gifts in the Netherlands, but was also surprisingly pleasant. After the long, drawn-out, freezing-cold Hunger Winter, I thought I'd hate everything to do with winter forever. I also thought I'd never again be happy. But a smile wreathed my face when I awoke in my warm bed on Christmas morning.

I climbed down to peer at Jan. "Hey, lazy bones, wake up. It's Christmas! Let's sneak down and see if the sisters decorated."

Jan didn't move; his eyes remained stubbornly shut.

Groaning, Trouble put his pillow over his head. "The decorations will still be there when it's light outside. Go back to sleep, Frits!"

It seemed I would have to do this without my usual partners in crime. After hurriedly putting on my clothes, I snuck out of the room. Even if the sisters had only put out one candle, I wanted to see it. I opened the playroom door slowly, careful that it wouldn't creak.

Silvery moonlight streamed through the net curtains, giving a magical feeling to the pine-scented room. Squinting my eyes to see better, I noticed an immense Christmas tree decorated with candles, red ribbons, and shiny ornaments standing in one corner. The sisters must have put it up last night. It would look amazing when they lit the candles!

I imagined everyone singing around the tree while I played Christmas carols on the piano. Oh, here comes Zuster Deenik, giving each of us a cup of hot chocolate. I could even taste it! Maybe there would be *een speculaasje*, too. My mouth filled with saliva.

"Frits! I thought I heard someone down here. What're you doing out of bed?" Zuster Dermout's piercing voice was thick with sleep.

The interruption of my daydream was so unexpected that coming up with a plausible lie was impossible. "Umm, well, I j…j…just wanted to see the decorations."

"Silly boy. Well, since you're up anyway, you can make a start on your chores. I'm going back to bed."

I frowned. I'd polished the brass, cleaned the shoes, and taken out the garbage yesterday. There was plenty of firewood, the *kachel* was glowing nicely, and I couldn't peel the potatoes so far in advance. What chore did the old bag want me to do? I cast my eyes around the room until they lit on the broken clock. I could fix that! I sat on the floor near the tree and got to work.

"*Kinderen*, come down for breakfast." Zuster Dermout called on her way down the stairs. She stopped at the door of the playroom. "What are you doing in here, Frits?"

"Umm, you told me I should do my chores, but they were all done. So, I fixed this clock. Look! It works now!"

"Hmmph. Silly child, always tinkering. Now it's time for breakfast."

Stung that she didn't admire and express gratitude for my achievement, rage bubbled up and exploded from my mouth. "I'm not silly! I bet you couldn't fix anything. That makes you silly. And stupid."

"Frits Evenblij! That's enough from you!" Zuster Dermout's brows pulled together.

"*Nee,* it's not. I fixed it! And now we know what time it is. Why are you so mean, Zuster Gemenerik?" My hands were on my hips.

"Are you talking back again? And what did you call me?" The sister's face was the color of a tomato.

Oops! I hadn't meant for all that to come out. I looked down and scuffed my shoe on the floor. "*Nee,* just explaining."

"Come over here!" Zuster Dermout indicated the wall behind her. "Stand facing it."

I shuffled toward her, blushing at the thought of everyone watching from their perches at the breakfast table.

"Hurry up!" Her voice was like nails on a blackboard. "Just here. You really must learn some respect."

After I was standing in place, Zuster Dermout hit me with the *mattenklopper* a "helpful" child brought her. Since I hadn't seen the blow coming, I lost my balance. My forehead and nose hit the wall, and blood cascaded down my shirt.

"Zuster Dermout," I began, holding my hand over my nose in a vain effort not to drip onto the floor. "I think…"

"That's the trouble with you. You always think you're right. Well, you're not. Learn now." She hit me again.

Tears springing to my eyes at what I perceived as yet another unjust beating, I clutched my chest and sank to the floor; the pain was almost unbearable.

Just then, Zuster Deenik came in. "Suus, I think perhaps Frits has learned his lesson. His mother will be here in a couple of days, you know. Let's just eat, shall we?"

Zuster Dermout raised her chin and sailed to the table to enjoy her Christmas breakfast.

Jan, who'd been watching our interchange with horrified eyes, came over and gently touched my forehead. "You have a gigantic lump there."

I shrugged. "It'll heal. Sit down and have some breakfast. I'll come sit by you soon."

But by the time I'd cleaned myself, the floor, and the wall, even with Zuster Deenik's help, no food was left. I seethed silently all the way through church.

Afterward, I stopped by where Zuster Dermout was darning socks.

"That was the last time. The last." I spoke through clenched teeth, my eyes shooting sparks.

Zuster Dermout looked up at me, and her eyes grew wide. I was far from taller than her, but with my broken nose, the lump on my forehead, and my clenched fists, I'm sure I looked tough. I meant to. After narrowing my eyes at her, I nonchalantly turned away and walked toward my friend.

"Hey man, you look terrible! What did you do?" It seemed Trouble had been more focused on food than on me during breakfast.

"Nothing except fix the clock," I whispered. "Zuster Gemenerik is an idiot, and I hate her. But she won't beat me again. Ever."

"We all hate her, but most of us know enough to stay out of her way." His wink and punch on my arm did much to diffuse the sting of those words, but not the next ones. "Anyway, I have great news."

"Oh yeah? Does Zuster Dermout have leprosy? Or maybe the plague?"

"*Nee,* it's nothing to do with her, you silly guy. It's me. Now that the war is over, and they've recovered a bit, my parents decided to take me out of *het kindertehuis.* I'm going to live with them and my brother in Amsterdam. I'm going home!"

My heart sank. Life without Trouble? It sounded unbearable.

"Wow. I'm happy for you. And for me, of course. You're such a pest!" I turned away so my friend wouldn't see my eyes turn red.

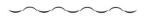

1946 Over the next few months, one by one, most of the children in *het kindertehuis* moved on, either to a boarding school or to live with their parents.

"When do you think Mama will have us come home? After all, if she doesn't have to pay for this place, she won't need to earn as much. And we're old enough to care for ourselves while she's at work."

"Don't hold your breath, Jan. As long as we're here, Mama can pretend she doesn't have *kinderen.* She doesn't love us, you know."

Jan shook his head. "*Nee,* you're wrong. Mothers always love their *kinderen.* She's just bad at showing her feelings."

I gazed at my brother's earnest little face. Could he be right? After all, Mama had sent us to an upper-class establishment. Maybe she actually did care. I decided to find out just how much when she came for a visit. But first, we had to get through the next few days.

"Frits, come here!" Zuster Dermout's lips were so stiff she could barely speak. "What do you mean by this?"

Pulling myself away from figuring out how to rewire a lamp, I followed her pointing finger. The shoes were clean and shiny, but I'd left the shoe polish out. I stifled a sigh. Honestly, what was her problem?

"I've told you time and time again. Do your chores before starting anything else. No half jobs."

I stood silent while staring her in the eyes, just waiting until she finished her rant. This time, I would not look down. I almost hoped she'd hit me so I could teach her a well-deserved lesson.

"And you can take that look off your face! I'll be speaking with your mother for sure."

Shrugging, I put away the polish and turned to leave the room. Her hand landed on my arm. An unwise move for sure! I immediately pried her fingers off me. Narrowing my eyes, I spoke slowly and clearly through clenched teeth. "Don't you ever touch me again!"

"Well, of all the disrespectful brats!" Zuster Dermout's voice was a continuous drone in my ears that grew fainter as I walked away. She did not follow me.

From that day forward, Zuster Dermout was often incensed with me, but she never hit me again. She found other ways to get even.

"Jan, have you been going through my things? I had my magnet and the slide rule from Papa in my cubbyhole, but just found them in this one."

"*Nee,* I know better than to touch your stuff!" Jan chuckled uneasily. Having polished up my temper, I no longer hesitated to use it.

"Well then, who?"

"Um, I saw Zuster Dermout over here earlier…"

Not waiting for my brother to finish, I stormed over to the sister, exploding before I even got near.

"You touched my stuff! What right do you have to go through my things?" I planted my feet apart, ready for anything.

Zuster Deenik jumped to her feet in alarm, but Zuster Dermout just looked at me over her glasses. "Whatever are you shouting about? Nothing here is yours. It's all on loan to you. If I want to go through your things, I will."

"My father gave me that slide rule! It's mine. Don't even think of saying it's not, you *gemenerik.*"

"Keep a civil tongue in your head, young man."

My vision clouded, and the blood pounded in my ears. "*Nee,* I won't. You're a stupid, ugly, old *teef* (b*tch)." I emphasized each word by ripping a flower out of the arrangement on the table and throwing it onto the floor.

A gentle hand on my back caused me to flinch and whirl around, fists clenched.

It was Juf van Kempen. "Frits, come on. Calm down. Let's go outside for a while."

I felt ashamed and stopped yelling—that time, anyway.

But, as the days went by, it became more and more difficult to cope with life. Even my beloved teacher seemed to be out to get me.

"Frits, this work is just not good enough. I know you'd rather be doing math or physics, but writing is an important part of your education. This is barely legible!"

I promised to do better but found it impossible to force myself to do anything other than precisely what I wanted to do. My grades in several classes went down. And when they did, I became too depressed and angry even to try to do better. My teacher and the sisters complained to Mama; the subsequent visit did not go well.

Dear Fritsje,

Now you can't say you had to wait a long time for a letter. It was not fun for you this time when I was in Driebergen, but that was your own fault. It wasn't fun for me either. And that was not my fault; therefore, it was much worse! But this is going to be the last time, isn't it, little boss? When I return, I hope we can both enjoy it, BOTH!

When I come again, it'll be your birthday. I hope we can celebrate a real, nice birthday, without complaints about the birthday boy. So, will you look after that, my boy?

You know there's more going on than a nice birthday. If you stay behind at school again, then you won't be allowed to be in the school photo. And if I get more complaints about your behavior, you won't be allowed to come to Den Haag in the summer! So be very sweet! But you promised me, and I want to trust your promise again!

Use your brain, sweetheart. You could have a lovely summer. You're allowed so much. You can join the Boy Scouts, do gym classes, ride your bike to Woestduin, etc. I'm really envying you! You need to tell me what you want for your birthday very soon. Make a list, but think a little about my purse!

Don't wait too long to write, or else I'll have so little time here to look for a present in a leisurely fashion. Let me especially know how it's going and if the sister is now satisfied with you. Goodbye, sweetheart. I still love you very much, so don't make me sad again!

Kisses, Mama

Once I finished reading this letter, I looked over at Jan, who was reading his letter. It was doubtless very different in tone from the one I'd received. She was correct; I'd promised to be good. But how could I? My insides churned perpetually.

Whenever Zuster Dermout looked at me, I remembered the many punishments, and my fists clenched. Whenever I was sent to the forest to collect wood, I remembered seeing dead bodies slung over a rosebush, and it became hard to breathe. When we went on an outing, I would remember Keetie and my cousins being taken away in the very same cart that was transporting the little ones. The war was over, but it was as if I was stuck in the stress of that time. My chest hurt, and relief only came from immersing myself in figuring out an electrical circuit, playing the piano, or stroking the soft fur of the home's pet dog. Being denied that I went ballistic.

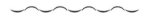

I was officially a teenager today, but Zuster Dermout saw no reason to celebrate. My elbows stuck out too far at breakfast as I cut my bread into the regulation squares. Zuster Dermout's solution, eating with a book in each armpit, made it very difficult to use utensils, but I had no choice. And I'd better finish the food!

Having caught the dragon's attention, she scrutinized my every move at lunch. Evidently, I committed the crime of briefly resting on my elbow, so she crept up and slammed it on the table. I jumped up with clenched fists, but remembering Mama's threats, swallowed hard and sat back down.

"*Nee,* Frits, to help you learn your lesson, eat the rest of your meal standing up."

Despite Zuster Dermout's best birthday efforts, I didn't lose it, but the required restraint made my chest hurt.

My impeccably dressed mother reeked of French perfume at her next visit, but she was no longer attractive in my eyes. Fury had consumed the joy and beauty in my life.

"Well, Frits, has your behavior improved?"

"I've been good enough," I mumbled.

"What did you say?"

Jan's eyes became saucers when I responded by shouting, "I'm doing fine. No thanks to you."

Mama took a deep breath and turned her back on me. "And Jan, how's your reading coming?"

My nostrils flared, and my face turned red. Jan often woke me with his recurrent nightmare: his teacher put him and a bear together in a large underground garbage can. It didn't take a genius to guess how he felt about school.

My brother really struggled with reading. I had no idea why and was infuriated that nobody, not his teacher nor the sisters or Mama, was helping.

"Leave him alone, Mama. It's not as if you care."

"Well, Frits, it looks like you won't be welcome in Den Haag this summer."

I shrugged. I wasn't sure I wanted to go, anyway. Here was better. Of course, Mama had threatened that she could deprive me of bicycling, swimming, and even joining the Boy Scouts. But I knew the sisters would be only too glad to get rid of the difficult boy. They wouldn't keep me inside.

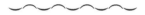

Diary entry, July 13, 1946

I woke up this morning, but I don't know why. I turned over and saw Sister standing in the opening of the door. She said, "Go back to sleep." I thought, *ja,* that's easy to say but not to do. I then tried to sleep, but it didn't happen. Then we got up. I got dressed and went downstairs.

I ate and then played a game with Appie and Marietta. I kept winning, no matter how much I tried to lose. Marietta was disappointed when I left. Then I looked up Bali with Hans and kept looking after he left.

Then I listened to the gramophone, and then I wrote in my diary. Everyone was looking at what I was writing, and I really didn't like that. I hated it that Marietta said she'd even read the whole thing. Liliane was super-annoying and kept trying to sit near me.

The weatherman said that tomorrow we will have thunderstorm panic in the middle of the country. I'm intrigued to know what that means.

Diary entry, January 3, 1947

I woke up this morning because Eddie pounded on the clothing rack. I grated cheese for breakfast before we ate, and then we ate. We were late because the sister's alarm was an hour late. After we had breakfast, we shoveled coal. I had an argument with Wim about who could shovel the anthracite the fastest. We will get the decision on January 5.

I was again an annoying boy because, instead of helping sister make up and clean the rooms, I played with my watches. Zuster Deenik called me, but I didn't know why. Then she asked me what all I'd done this morning. I said that I shoveled coal and played with my watches. She said, "Fine."

Then I went downstairs and decided to help her to clean the rooms. In the afternoon, I washed the windows in the entire house and got 10 cents in pay. I gave it to Jan because he's saving to buy Mama some knives. She only has two. I was allowed to stay up until eight and then I went to bed.

Diary entry, January 4, 1947

This morning, I again wiped the windows in the conservatory, kitchen, glass cabinet, and hall door. I also chopped wood in our forest. In the afternoon, I chopped wood in the forest near the church on the Melvill van Carnbeelaan and Beaufortlaan.

Then I went with Tante Toors and Zuster Dermout to the Bochove's house to get apples. They were almost all frozen. Then we had to get undressed, but I had to get dressed again to go to the pharmacist, van de Meene. We always have to get undressed early on Saturday nights because that's when our clothing is put in the laundry.

Another year had passed at *het kindertehuis*. The sisters were no longer stressed out by caring for too many children because Jan, Jantje, Wim, Eddie, and I were the only young inhabitants left. They were strict but now also displayed a modicum of kindness. I developed a grudging affection for my two caretakers, even though I knew I could never behave well enough for them to feel any actual affection for me. Jan was also unloved, being far too withdrawn to elicit warm feelings. No matter. The lack didn't bother us. As Jan told me in a philosophical moment, if a person has no recollection of having ever received a hug, that person doesn't miss them.

We were strangely content with our daily lives. With so few people in the home, there were hardly any chores. More time for bicycling, playing in the forest, and listening to music. There was also more food, which growing boys always enjoy. We were settled. Almost.

There was one dream we both held close to our hearts: to live at home like normal children do. When the sisters announced they were closing *het kindertehuis*, we hoped our dream would finally come true.

Frits's earlier diary entries,1945. (top)

Frits and Jan at the swimming "pool" in Woestduin in Doorn, 1946. Note how emaciated Frits still is. (bottom)

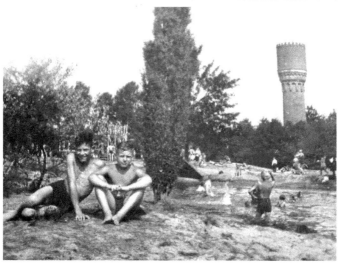

9

THE REJECTION

The sun streamed through the window to the playroom, where we'd been waiting since breakfast. I'd checked and rechecked our bedroom and cubbies. *Ja*, all we possessed was in the two small *koffers* sitting at our feet. For me, the case was infinitely more valuable than the contents— because of who it had belonged to.

Zuster Deenik took a seat next to me. "So, it's the end of your time here. We've been through a lot together, both good and bad. I do hope you'll remember us with affection as we'll remember you."

I chuckled. "Maybe you will, but I'm sure Zuster Dermout won't."

"Oh, Frits, it was her responsibility to bring you up to be a gentleman. You're not there yet, but she gave you a good start."

I rolled my eyes. "Whatever you say…"

"And you, Jan? Will you remember us?"

I held my breath. When Jan offered no response except to mumble, "Maybe Mama will let us stay up past 8:00," I blew it out.

Jan hated the sisters passionately. Watching me being abused had been more painful for him than being beaten had been for me. He was not about to forgive.

"Oh look, Mama's here!" I exclaimed, perhaps more enthusiastically than was warranted.

Jan peered out the window. "Who's that old man with her? Do you know?"

"No idea. Maybe someone to help with the luggage? Or a Dutch houseboy?" I shrugged.

Jan chuckled. "I doubt he could lift a book, let alone a *koffer*."

Mama came through the door with a swish of her skirts. "*Goedemiddag*, Zuster Deenik." She turned to us. "Oh, Frits and Jan, I

150

see you're ready. Good. We'll go as soon as I settle up with the sisters." Mama paused for breath and then drew the tall, bald man standing slightly behind her forward. "But first, let me introduce you to your new father, Meneer Jacobus Ouwerkerk."

"What? When? Why d...d...didn't we know?" I turned red, hearing my words tumbling over each other. I stuffed my hands in my pockets to stop their twirling. Jan stood by; his silence was almost audible.

Mama frowned. "Frits, *doe maar gewoon*, but also take your hands out of your pockets." She continued, "We got married a few months ago. It wasn't worth bothering you with it then. Now, shake hands nicely with Vader."

Jan stepped forward and mutely offered the man his rather grubby paw. I put mine behind my back.

"He's not my father," I muttered.

Mama sighed. "Why do you always have to be so difficult?"

Vader cleared his throat. "Frits..." he began ponderously.

Mama shook her head. "Not now, Cobus."

After a silent journey, we arrived at their apartment in Den Haag. It looked very similar to our former home, with much of the same kind of furniture, ornaments, and rugs on the tables. Seeing the imprint of my own Papa's head in his slightly scorched chair forced me to blink back childish tears.

"Bring your *koffers* up to the room on the left for now. But don't unpack them. Frits, you'll move to Concordia College, the boarding school in Emmastraat, on Monday. We found you a school in Den Haag."

I shrugged. I hadn't set my hopes on living at home, anyway. As long as Jan could, I'd be satisfied. But Mama wasn't finished.

"Jan, you're too young for Concordia College, so you'll live with a foster family in Scheveningen and take the tram to a school in Den Haag."

Jan grew pale. "But Mama, I thought I'd live with you and attend a school nearby!"

"Ridiculous! We're newlyweds. We can't have boys living here. The foster family has a son who's your age—it's an ideal situation. We'll take you there tomorrow so you have time to settle in before you start school."

The pain in Jan's eyes caused steam to leak from my ears. An explosion quickly followed. "That's inexcusable! What kind of mother are you? Jan has been living without parents since he was two. Two!

151

The poor kid was hoping he might be like everyone else and live with his mother, but you're sending him away again!"

Vader cleared his throat, but I ignored him. "What did Jan ever do to you that you treat him like this? I'm the difficult one—so you say, anyway. Jan has only ever been good. But you, you're not just unloving and selfish. You're wicked, too! You disgust me."

Mama gasped and fell back onto the chaise lounge. Her new husband, puffing out his chest, stepped forward to place himself between his bride and her eldest son.

Sneering, I pinned the wannabe hero with my eyes. "I'm sorry for you being married to her. I never thought I'd think this, but Papa and Meneer Goudsmit were lucky to die. They escaped her clutches. You won't."

Vader, who I was to learn, did everything at a snail's pace, again cleared his throat, and opened his mouth, but I didn't wait for more. I ran out the door, slamming it behind me.

After rushing down the street with tears streaming down my face and rain soaking my hair, I stopped on a bridge. It was time to make some decisions about my future.

First, since my success was solely up to me, I'd make sure that I worked hard. In the past, I'd let my schoolwork slide, more because I didn't care than because I couldn't do it. That would end today. I would do so well that if Mama told anyone I was difficult, she'd be proven a liar. And more importantly, one day, I would achieve my dream of being an engineer.

My eyes narrowed as I recalled all the ways in which Mama had disappointed me. She acted nothing like any other mother I knew. What could I do about that? With a quick nod, I decided. This woman would no longer be my mama. I couldn't disown her completely, but from this day forward, she would be "Moeder." Technically, she was the one who'd given birth to me, but she'd never again be anything more.

Finally, even though the sermon sometimes played on my mind, I decided I would never forgive her. Never. She didn't deserve it. That day, I added several layers to the wall around my heart.

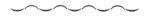

With my hands on my hips, I grinned while watching Jan bounce on his over-stuffed *koffer*. "I think you have everything you'll need, Jan. It's not as if you're moving to another country."

Jan's blue eyes remained dry, but his sigh came from his toes.

"Boys, it's time to go," Vader called from the front door.

"Can't wait to get rid of us!" I muttered so only Jan could hear.

Vader, Moeder, Jan, and I took Tram 11 to its terminus and then walked the short distance to Jan's foster home. Living into his role as the patriarch, Vader pompously cleared his throat before ringing the bell. I turned around to observe our surroundings while we waited for the door to be opened. The row house was near the promenade, the pier, and the sea. As I squinted into the sun, it looked to me as if the lighthouse would be visible from the front window. I was cautiously hopeful that this place wouldn't be too bad for my pre-teen brother.

A tall woman in an apron and kerchief opened the door. "*Goedemorgen* Meneer and Mevrouw Ouwerkerk. *Alstublieft* come in." She graced us with a snaggle-toothed smile before calling up the stairs, "Pieter, come down and meet your new roommate."

I pulled Jan out from behind me and gently shoved him through the door. He'd never had a special friend at *het kindertehuis*. Perhaps now he would. With a wry grin, I whispered, "Go on. It couldn't be more unpleasant than living with Vader and Moeder."

Jan's round blue eyes and tight shoulders told me he feared it might be worse. But the sooner he got over the idea that I was his protector, the better. It would no longer be possible for me to be with him every day.

Mevrouw Schevetanden, who had to go up the stairs to convince her son to come down, came into the room holding an equally reluctant Pieter's elbow. "There now. See, Pieter, Jan isn't so bad. And this is his *broer*, Frits."

Pieter twisted his mouth into a passable imitation of a grin, revealing a gap between his two front teeth. I stared, fascinated with his red hair, which stood on end like he'd put his finger in an electric socket. Jan had some experience with that!

"Now, you boys all go on up to Pieter's room. Pieter, show Jan his bed and where to put his clothing while the grown-ups have a cup of tea."

"Come on, Jan and, uh, Frits, is it? I have a bunk bed, you know. Jan will have the top, and I'll have the bottom." Well, he sounded friendly enough.

Following Pieter while dragging my brother by the hand, I wrinkled my nose and glanced at Jan. Had he noticed the pungent, moldy smell, which grew stronger as we ascended? Jan shrugged. Sometimes we could communicate without words. I would miss that.

Oblivious to our silent exchange, Pieter continued chattering. "You know, Mamma said we have to let you live here because your mother will pay. With Pappa gone, we could use a bit extra. That's okay, I guess, but I really don't need a *broer*. You see, I have mice."

I looked to where Pieter was pointing and noticed a white mouse. It was fearlessly grooming its whiskers while sitting on Pieter's bed. There was another on his chest of drawers. Worse, there were what appeared to be little brown grains of rice liberally sprinkled on the blanket and all along the edges of the floor. I looked closer. They even covered most surfaces. Jan's eyes grew wider as he, too, saw the free-range mice—and their droppings.

"Um, don't you keep them in a cage?"

"Oh, *nee,* they're much happier when allowed to roam around. Such sweet little creatures. They get everywhere. I've found them in my bed, the heating pipes, and even my shoes. It's so cute!"

I shook my head, took a deep breath through my mouth, and shrugged. I didn't envy Jan living with the mice, but there were worse things. Like living with Moeder.

Just then, we heard the rumbling and squeal of a tram. Jan ran to the window. "Look, Frits, it goes right by here!" Driebergen was too small for a tram, so this was new and exciting for my brother.

Pieter puffed up his chest. "Yup. You'll take that tram to your school every day—and home every night. It's easy on the way back since you get off at the terminus. You'll have to watch for your stop on the way there."

"Won't you be going with me?" Jan's voice was small.

"*Nee,* your mother selected a school in the city center of Den Haag. My mamma wondered why because there's a perfectly good school near here. She said it's probably something to do with you being a spoiled rich kid."

I raised my eyebrows. Spoiled? Rich? Try neglected, a cast-off in every way. I opened my mouth.

"Where's the school?" My brother trembled visibly, forcing me to intervene instead of setting his new roommate straight.

"Don't worry, Jan. You can just count the stops and get off at the right number. You'll be fine."

"Jan and Frits, come down. Vader and I are going now." Moeder's carefully modulated voice only just carried up the stairs. She was clearly putting on a show.

We clomped down to find her and Vader already in their coats. Vader handed mine to me. Moeder turned to Jan and offered him her cool cheek, which he dutifully kissed. "Goodbye, Jan. Be good." Vader shook his hand and said the same.

I stood back, watching my brother's carefully emotionless face, my heart breaking. Then I punched him in the arm. "Chin up, Jan. We'll write, okay?"

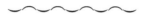

Moeder and Vader's apartment was quiet over the next few days, and it was entirely due to my seething presence. I answered questions with as few words as possible and never initiated a conversation. Sometimes, I pretended I hadn't heard Vader speak. Better to avoid engaging with him. Moeder didn't even try. If at all possible, I rode Vader's bicycle to make myself scarce, did a jigsaw to distract myself from Jan's situation, or tinkered with electronics. Just because I loved doing that. Finally, the day came when they could dispose of the other son--me.

This time, Vader, Moeder, and I took the bus to Emmastraat in the Bezuidenhout neighborhood of Den Haag. The bombed-out buildings took me back to the many nights when I cowered under my blanket, frightened that an Allied bomb would hit *het kindertehuis.* The difference here was that this bombing had been a stupid mistake. I remembered Juf van Kempen telling us that someone in the Royal Air Force had reversed the negatives before telling the pilots where to set the coordinates! The error led to 67 bombs being dropped on a residential neighborhood overcrowded with evacuees, killing over 500 people. It also destroyed mementos of the only part of my childhood where I was happy.

After a short walk, we reached a large, burgundy brick house.

"Here we are. Concordia College for boys." Vader's overly loud voice suggested he was trying to diffuse the oppressive atmosphere.

Not going to work. I climbed the outside stairs ahead of Moeder, my *koffer* in hand. "Okay, goodbye then."

Moeder exhaled noisily. "Frits, stop being so very difficult. We'll be going in with you. The principal will expect that."

I rolled my eyes. "How strange for him to expect a parent actually to be concerned about her child. Just imagine that! But you must, of course, keep up appearances."

Vader's heavy hand came down on my shoulder, ensuring that I wouldn't continue my diatribe and embarrass them in front of the faculty. Moeder rang the bell, and a gray-haired woman in a black dress and white apron opened the ornately carved wooden doors. I was later to learn that she was the housemother, Juffrouw Verwaand.

"Ah, you must be Meneer and Mevrouw Ouwerkerk. And you're Frits?"

"Yes, I'm Frits Evenblij." I emphasized my last name before pointing at Vader. "He's not my father."

Vader's fingers dug into my shoulder, eliciting a gasp of pain.

Juf Verwaand's eyebrows drew together. "Of course, of course, come in, come in. Follow me. I'll seat you and then check if Meester Fretgezicht is free."

Her high heels clacked on the tile floor as she led us to a large office with a massive desk and leather chair on one side and three hardback chairs on the other. The front window behind us was covered in net curtains and framed in heavy red and gold brocade drapes. I perched on the edge of the chair furthest from the door while Moeder sat in the middle chair, and Vader sat furthest from me. Moeder patted her hair into place, arranged her skirt just so, delicately crossed her legs at the ankles, and peeled off her gloves.

I rolled my eyes at her ostentatious preparations but then retreated into my head. What would this place be like? Would Juf Verwaand or Meester Fretgezicht try to beat me, "try" being the operative word? Would they have the same ridiculous rules as *het kindertehuis*? I'd had enough of following orders! I deliberately unclenched my fists—time to think of something else.

A painting of happy children, some dressed and some naked, graced the wall behind the headmaster's desk. That was weird, but I knew artists sometimes painted things that sure wouldn't happen in real life. My attention was drawn by a couple of boys with their heads together, just like Trouble and me when hatching a plot. Would I make any friends here? A girl in a blue dress sat reading under a tree, apparently oblivious to the children cavorting around her. She was focused. I'd vowed to do well academically, but what if the work was too difficult? What if I could only learn under the guidance of Juf van Kempen?

My stomach rose into my throat and made it difficult to breathe. Recognizing the onset of panic, I closed my eyes and remembered the words of the hymn. "Whatever the future may bring, the Lord's hand is leading me; To the place that he's preparing…" Even though I doubted the existence of God, my pulse slowed.

Finally, finally, the door opened to admit a slight gentleman whose face reminded me of the rodents that graced my brother's new bedroom. Vader immediately rose to his feet. Moeder gave me a look, so I reluctantly got up, as well. I wanted to prove that anything she might say or had said about me was wrong.

"Sit down, sit down," Meester Fretgezicht invited, taking his seat behind the desk. I suppressed a chuckle. Was it a rule here that a person had to say everything twice?

The headmaster gazed at me, his squinty eyes lingering on my face and then my bare legs. In those days, boys didn't wear long pants until they were 15, which was still half a year away. I wished it wasn't.

Vader cleared his throat to prepare to talk—glacially, of course.

Moeder, in the interim, jumped in with her typical formalities. "*Dank u wel*, Meester Fretgezicht, for taking Frits now, part way through the school year. The closure of *het kindertehuis* in Driebergen put us in an unfortunate position."

"That's fine, that's fine. We've heard good things about that place. We're happy to provide him with a place to live. We understand he'll attend the Maatschappij tot het Nut van het Algemeen School (NUTS). It's a shame you can't afford classes here, but the NUTS school is a good alternative. We're sure it will further advance your son's education, and you'll be very satisfied. Now, do you wish to tour the home, or do you have other plans?"

During this speech, I found it hard not to burst out laughing. Why was the headmaster using the royal "we?" Anyone could see he was alone here!

Moeder stood up so Vader could help her into her coat. "No need for a tour. We'll take our leave now and entrust Frits into your capable hands, Meester Fretgezicht." She offered me her cheek, but I pretended not to notice.

Once they'd sailed out the front door, Meester Fretgezicht smoothed his oily hair before indicating that I should accompany him on a tour of the house: three schoolrooms, a refectory with long tables, and ward-style bedrooms. All pretty standard. That is until he led me to the large back garden, which had, of all things, a coop with six white leghorn chickens. Watching them diligently pecking the soil in their search for grubs brought forth my first genuine smile in many days. I'd loved visiting the farms near Driebergen.

"Chickens! In Den Haag!" I sputtered.

"*Ja, ja.* We expect all our young charges to help with gardening, harvesting food, collecting eggs, and general chores. We're sure you'll get used to it. *Ja zeker*, you'll get used to it." Meester Fretgezicht's smile revealed a mouthful of crooked yellow teeth, but at least it reached his eyes. I was silent for a moment while deciding how best to respond. Well, it wasn't his fault that he was born ugly, and I did want to do well at this school.

"*Bedankt, bedankt.*" I hesitated to see if he'd noticed the repetition before continuing. "I'll be happy to do chores like I did at *het kindertehuis*. I'm especially g...g...good at fixing electronics. So, if you have any broken radios, clocks, watches..." I looked up hopefully.

Meester Fretgezicht's tiny eyes sparkled. "Hmm, it's not exactly gardening, but still a useful, if unusual, skill set. We'll bear it in mind. Now, let's introduce you to the other boys."

So began my time at Concordia College. I didn't find friends since everyone else went to school here. But at least we weren't at war, and the *mattenklopper* was kept where it belonged: with the cleaning supplies. I grudgingly conceded that this place was okay. Even Jan didn't appear to be suffering in his foster home—well, not too badly, anyway.

Dear Frits,

This place is berserk! Every night, I'm woken by mice scurrying across my face. Pieter refuses to keep them in their cage. I can't complain because he hates me enough already. Who knows? If I said anything, he might decide to keep pet cockroaches.

The first day of school was hard. There I stood by myself in front of a new school with a playground full of children. But I acted brave like you taught me, and I did it. You would be proud of how I still strut like a peacock, even though I don't have any friends.

Guess what? My teacher is nice. He even taught me how to draw a tree with branches and leaves. I put the drawing under my mattress where the mice can't chew on it. I don't know what cockroaches eat.

Please write. I hope to see you soon.

Your artistic brother, Jan

I read this letter twice, chuckling at my brother's signature sense of humor. His way with words was kind of like mine with electronics. How odd that he struggled so much with reading! On the other hand, Jan having no friends didn't surprise me. He'd grown more and more withdrawn while at *het kindertehuis*. I'd overheard an adult in Driebergen saying that the experiences of Jan's life might have rendered him incapable of having a relationship with anyone apart from me. I hoped they were wrong because I wasn't there.

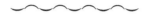

1948 A few months later, Jan joined me at Concordia College. Neither of us knew why he had to leave the foster home, but he laughingly assured me he wasn't sorry to be rid of Pieter and his mice. His special jobs here would be to feed and water the chickens, collect the eggs, and clean the coop. I wasn't convinced his situation had improved. Chickens are stinky! Still, I hoped this place would be as good for him as it was for me.

The days were growing longer, but the temperature was still frigid. I woke with my covers pulled up to my chin and my feet like blocks of ice. But it was the stench that commanded my attention. What was it? It smelled like…urine! Adjusting my blanket so my feet were covered and could defrost, I propped myself up on my elbow and whispered as loudly as I dared, "Hey Jan! Wake up. Can you smell that?"

Jan's eyes popped open. "That's not funny, Frits! I'll get in trouble," he hissed.

"Wha…?"

"My bed. You poured water in it…oh…oh, no!" Jan unpeeled himself from his sodden sheets and wailed, "I wet the bed!"

"So, the smell was you!" I quickly went into big brother mode. "Don't worry—we can fix it. Go now and get washed and dressed before anyone else wakes up. I'll let Juffrouw Verwaand know. She's nice. It'll be okay."

Even in the semi-darkness, I could see my brother's face get red as he mumbled, "I'm nearly 12! What an idiot I am!"

"Never mind, Jan. These things happen."

Later that day, I saw the newly washed sheets hanging out to dry and turned to look at Jan. He pretended not to notice them, but I could read his face. He was mortified. On the positive side, even though the bedwetting continued, no one there ever made him feel worse about it than he already did. If they had, I would've ensured they never did it again! But I wondered why Jan should begin wetting the bed now.

"Hey, Jan. What's going on with you? Are you unhappy here?"

Jan shook his head. "*Nee,* not really. Meester Fretgezicht looks like a rat, but he's nice. He's helping me with my lessons. He says I'm behind because I've been to so many schools, but I think maybe I'm just stupid. Anyway, he seems to like me. Sometimes, he even has me sit on his lap."

My eyes narrowed as my radar began humming. "Um, what? That's not really normal, Jan. In fact, it's creepy!"

"It is? He doesn't hurt me. It feels weird when he strokes my legs, but..." Jan shrugged it off.

I did not. I'd heard about men who prey on boys and was determined that my undersized brother shouldn't be a victim. From then on, whenever possible, I hung around when Jan was with Meester Fretgezicht.

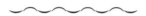

1949 "Frits, your tongue is sticking out again."

"Leave me alone, Jan. I'm busy."

"Whatcha doing?" Jan leaned over me as I scribbled in my diary.

"Just recording what I did today. I made a plug, switches, and a lock for the door. It's so cool that they let me do all those things."

Jan laughed and pointed at my cheek. "You forgot to write that you painted the railing. At least, your black cheek suggests you did. Maybe you should write that you painted your face and the railing."

I swatted his hand away. "Come on, *jongeman*. It's time for dinner."

"Mmm, it smells good, too."

We dropped into our seats and, after the mandatory grace, began eating. I started with my favorite, the liver, while Jan saved his favorite, the potato, until last. I'd discovered this difference between us when, thinking I was doing him a favor, I swiped what remained on his plate, and he objected.

"Jan, your father is here. Come down. Come down." Juffrouw Verwaand came bustling into the dining hall.

I swiped my hand across my mouth before scowling, "He's not our father."

She didn't hear me, but Jan did.

"Yeah, I know, I know," Jan answered me with a twinkle in his eyes. "Still, he is here, is here."

Noticing nobody was following her, Juf Verwaand returned to where we were still sitting. "Come on, Jan!"

He got up to go with her, and I came after him, a few steps behind.

"Not you, not you, Frits. Your father only wants Jan to come."

This was so strange that I forgot to protest. Why would Vader fetch Jan but not me? And where were they going? Had they found him another foster home?

Once Vader and Jan departed, I asked, but Juf Verwaand didn't answer. Meester Fretgezicht wasn't there, so I couldn't ask him either. With rounded shoulders, I got up to wash the dishes.

"Where do you think ol' Fretgezicht is?" came a whisper from the walk-in pantry.

I slowed my hands to lessen the clinking of the crockery, straining to overhear.

"I bet they caught him. I sure hope so."

"What do you mean? Caught him? Is he a thief?"

"No. Worse. Do you ever hear the little boys crying at night?"

"Yeah, but when I told Juf Verwaand, she said they're just homesick. She refused to even check on them."

"Well, maybe it's not that. Did you see the painting in his office? And have you ever noticed how he always has a kid on his lap?"

Connecting the dots, I gasped. Unfortunately, when the speakers noticed I'd overheard, they closed the pantry door.

That night, I lay in bed worrying. I was grateful that, usually, Jan slept in the same room as me, but I still didn't know where he was now. I didn't trust Vader. What if he was like Meester Fretgezicht? My brow furrowed. Vader had been over 50 years old when he married Moeder, and I knew he'd never been married before. So, what was going on there? I got very little sleep.

Jan came back to Concordia College late the following afternoon, and I quickly drew him aside.

"Where were you? Why did you have to go with Vader?"

Jan shook his head. "It was so strange. Vader took me to court, where a judge asked me all about Meester Fretgezicht."

"What did he want to know?"

"Oh, he asked if Meester Fretgezicht ever visited me at night and if he ever touched me."

A chill went through me. "Did he?"

"Only what I told you. Sometimes, he had me sit on his lap. That's all."

"What about Vader? Did he hurt you?"

"*Nee,* of course not! You're so odd sometimes!"

Meester Fretgezicht did not return to the school; he'd been arrested and convicted of being much too fond of little boys. Within the month, Concordia College was disbanded.

As we packed, Jan and I speculated about where we would be placed next. We both knew it was only a matter of time before Moeder got rid of us. Again.

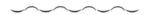

It was a blustery day in June when Vader escorted us to Charlotte de Bourbonstraat 130, a sparkling new red brick rowhouse. I craned my neck to look up at the arched windows of the three-story building with its ornately carved front doors, each with its own brass bell pull. Moeder always wanted to appear as patrician as her self-important mother, and I expected this place of residence would more than satisfy her.

It didn't, and we heard the complaints from dawn until dusk. If I'd liked him, I might have felt sorry for Vader. The neighborhood was not to her satisfaction, being near the Station Hollands Spoor and the Schenkviaduct. Even worse, the neighbors were working class. In her opinion, that was beneath contempt. She certainly wouldn't be making any friends here!

"Frits, Jan, come help with making dinner." As always, Vader's voice made the hair stand up on the back of my neck.

Moeder was lying on the chaise lounge right next to Papa's chair. With my eyes half-closed, I stuffed my hands in my pockets and slouched against the living room wall. "Why should I? I want to work on building a better radio. What's wrong with Moeder's hands?"

Jan bit his bottom lip. "Come on, Frits. Let's just do it."

"You help. You can take the old man's orders, but not me. Never. He's not my father." I shrugged one shoulder, but my fists clenched.

"Did you have something to say, Frits?" Vader came out of the kitchen, while carefully drying his hands.

If he meant to intimidate me, I would soon show him how well that would work. I'd been to hell and back and certainly wasn't afraid of a ponderous old man. "Yup. I said that I don't like you and won't take your orders. In fact, I'm going out."

"Oh, let him go, Cobus. I have a headache and can do without the shouting," came a faint voice from the chaise lounge.

162

"Ha! My shouting? What about your ridiculous faking? I'm so sick of you, lying there thinking you're special when you're the worst mother in the world!"

"Frits!" Vader now stood with his hands on his hips.

My lips pressed together, I made a rude gesture before leaving and slamming the door as hard as possible. Even though it was raining, I walked up the Schenkviaduct. There, I looked down and watched the large round discs turning whenever the locomotives had to face a different direction. How did they work? I closed my eyes, imagining what was happening inside the discs.

As my temper gradually cooled, I realized I would also have to change direction if I didn't want to crash. My current trajectory would doubtless lead to living somewhere other than home, possibly without my more compliant brother. That might be better for me, but it would be worse for him. And maybe for me, too.

To live at home, my ongoing rage would need to be pushed down deep where it would never see the light of day. I struggled with bundling up and stuffing the unwieldy creature, even as it reminded me of Jan's face when Moeder left him in foster care. Smoke came out of my nostrils as the monster harked back to the fact that Moeder had been on vacation when Papa died. My eyes filled with tears as it whispered that I shouldn't even be alive. After all, my cousins and Keetie were dead—I'd only escaped because Moeder consistently ignored her heritage. Everywhere I looked, rage showed me a self-centered woman, and I didn't like her at all. But she was my mother. I drew her face in the gravel and ground it into sand before deciding to do my best to put up with the person I called Moeder.

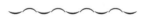

It was well after dark when I finally walked to the house, pulled the door open, and crept into the bedroom I shared with my brother. Jan was tossing and turning, every so often letting out a moan. Being well acquainted with nightmares, I grasped his shoulder to shake him awake. Oh, no! He was hot, burning up with fever! Could the dysentery have returned? I sniffed cautiously. Didn't seem like it.

When I called her, Moeder came to the bedroom to assess whether it was necessary to call a doctor. Jan was experiencing aches, pains, fever, and no appetite, but she deemed his life wasn't at risk. She told me to give him sips of water and administer aspirin.

A few days later, the mystery was solved. Every day for three days, more and more itchy bumps appeared; Jan had chicken pox and was totally miserable.

Moeder made a flying visit to our bedroom: to instruct him not to scratch. After all, it would be terrible to have a son with unsightly scars! She then took a seat on the chaise lounge and began writing her next novel.

It was Vader who brought Jan, who was pitifully grateful for any and all attention, hot drinks and tidbits of food.

"It itches so much!" Jan frantically rubbed a particularly large vesicle.

Vader, who had been sitting on the side of Jan's bed stroking his hair, nodded. "I'll be back." A few minutes later, he appeared, laden with cotton wool and a bottle of calamine lotion.

"This should help, Jan. Take off your pajamas, and I'll put this on all your bumps. It'll stop the itch."

I glared at Vader as Jan obediently removed his pajamas. Ignoring me, Vader put lotion on a cotton ball and applied it everywhere on Jan's body.

I waited, pretending to be absorbed in my crossword until Vader finished his ministrations. Once he closed the door, I verbally accosted my brother. "Jan, what are you thinking? That's just bizarre! He's not your real father, and you're allowing him to do things even Moeder wouldn't do."

"She never does anything, and he's helping me," Jan mumbled, his arms over his face.

"It's weird and way too close to what Meester Fretgezicht is serving time for. Just put the lotion on yourself."

Jan sighed. "Frits, I understand you hate him, but I don't. He's the first person ever, besides you, to be kind to me. He's not creepy, and I love him."

Discussing Vader with my brother seemed pointless, but I wasn't about to let the subject drop. The next evening, I watched to see when Vader would go in for a repeat performance. After giving them 10 minutes, I burst into the room. "Get your hands off him, you sick man! You disgust me."

"What are you talking about, Frits? Jan is itchy; I'm helping him."

"Does Moeder know what you are? About what you're doing?" My entire body trembled, and the onerous responsibility to protect Jan overwhelmed me.

"Out!" Vader's eyes were blazing as he pointed to the bedroom door. Seeing Jan was nearly asleep, I backed away. After all, I definitely wouldn't be able to guard my brother if I no longer lived here. But what could I do if Jan didn't want what I was offering?

"Frits, Jan, come and have a quick look here." Moeder was napping again, so Vader spoke in a low voice. His leering mouth did nothing to complement his sparkling eyes. Confused, we followed him into the living room, past Moeder, to where he hid behind the kitchen drapes and pointed. There, across the backyards, curtains open, a young lady was bathing herself at her kitchen sink. Her bottom and a breast were clearly visible. Being 16 years old, my cheeks turned red, but I had a good look. After all, this was the first naked, fully grown woman I'd ever seen. Jan's reaction was quite different. He shrugged. "What's for dinner?"

Later that day, while repairing the neighbor boy's toy train, I thought about what happened. Why was an old man like Vader staring at an unclothed neighbor? He was married! And why did he point her out to my 14-year-old brother? My fists clenched.

Naturally, my animosity toward Vader led to problems. Fiery anger boiled over regularly, escalating into shouting matches that drew the attention of our neighbors. Eventually, Vader had enough.

"Rita, you need to choose. Him or me. One of us has to go."

It was me. With a wry grin, I reflected that I'd known it was a matter of time. Moeder put up no argument and quickly found me a barely furnished and unheated room at the Barentszstraat 57. She paid the nominal rent only because working during high school was forbidden. No provision was made for clothing, and I ate what little my host family provided. My pants and sleeves became shorter and shorter as I grew in height but not width. I was now 5'10" tall and 139 pounds soaking wet.

But, and this was extremely important to me, I was finally free. My landlord couldn't care less what I did with my time, so I went where I wanted when I wanted. The only one who set rules was me. Once my schoolwork was done, I could swim around the pier, walk in a park, or ride the old bicycle Moeder provided so I could get to the NUTS school. I never had to hear Vader's tiresome tones or Moeder's languid requests. I didn't even have to protect my brother, who remained at home. We were back to writing letters.

I enjoyed the fascinating school excursions; my classes (except for German) held my attention, and my grades were mostly good. I even collected a small group of friends who readily joined in with the adventures I dreamed up. One friend, Henk, soon became a bosom pal because he shared my fascination with all things electronic.

Meanwhile, my family moved to the Statenkwartier: the van Hoornbeekstraat off the Prins Mauritslaan. Jan wrote that they now lived in an upstairs apartment where they shared the front door and hall with another family. Apparently, Moeder liked it better there because the area was more aristocratic—in her eyes, anyway. I hoped Jan would be happier now, especially since he was living in the absence of the turmoil my presence always caused. He wasn't.

Dear Frits,

Well, I just started in my fourth school this year. I'm the oldest and the dumbest kid in my class. In fact, my teacher, Meneer van Stijn, has me sit at the back of the classroom so I can do what he thinks I'm fit for: refill the coal stove.

I had one friend, Lotte, who lives across the balcony from us. Since her parents aren't home after school either, she invited me to her house to make pancakes. The problem is her dad got mad about me being there when he wasn't home. We didn't do anything, not even make pancakes! He complained to Mama, so I can't go again. No more friend.

A man who owns the garage below us noticed I'm alone a lot and let me sit in his old car. That was fun, but Meester van Stijn saw me and objected. I'm not sure why. Maybe he wants to make sure I'm always lonely.

Are you sad yet? Let me cheer you up. Vader bought me a black Fongers bike! Now I can come and visit you.

Your bicycling brother, Jan

Henk looked up from where he was wiring the transmitter for a ham radio. Our goal was to be able to talk to each other outside of school, and we were close to achieving it.

"Hey, Frits, did you see the advertisement on the bulletin board at the post office?"

"Which one?"

"I saw it yesterday. There's a farmer in de Woude who's looking for summer help. It sounds like the kind of thing you'd enjoy—mucking out chickens and taking care of cows."

"Ha! Judging by your screams and clucks as you jumped off the pier, I think you'd be more at home with the chickens. For me, just give me bulls. I haven't tried bull riding, but I'm sure it'd be fun."

Henk took in my sparsely decorated room. "Well, have a look next time you go. It'd be a lot better than living here. I don't know how you stand it! And you could earn some pocket money. Maybe replace those pants…"

I shook my head. "Forget the pants. A job would enable me to pay some of my rent and hopefully stop Moeder from complaining so much. Honestly, she's more generous to her cat, Poemel, than me!"

"So, do you think you'll apply?"

"Oh, yes. Definitely." I rocked back in my chair and put my hands behind my head, my eyes unfocused. "Working in a tiny village surrounded by water on all four sides would make for an amazing summer."

Crash! Henk snickered as I picked myself up from the floor.

I threw a pencil at him. "And if you finish your radio, we can even talk while I'm there!"

I applied and got the job. After the school year ended, I cycled to the tiny wooden ferry that crossed the wide channel to de Woude. A wizened man accepted my money, and with the fragrant wind ruffling my hair, I breathed deeply and leaned on the railing.

"First time visiting de Woude, *jongeman*?"

"*Ja*, I'm going to be working here for the summer. But tell me, is it true that this entire village is surrounded by water?"

"Yup! De Woude will never grow because it's bordered by two lakes: the Alkmaardermeer and the Uitgeestermeer. And we love it that way."

"I'm looking forward to exploring it."

"Won't take you long," chuckled the elderly man as he docked the ferry and opened the gate to let me off.

Grabbing my bike, I crossed the street and rang the village's combination hotel and restaurant's doorbell.

"Can I help you?"

"*Ja*, I'm Frits Evenblij. I wrote to book a room for a night. I'll be starting work tomorrow."

"Of course," the lady said while wiping her hands on her apron. "Welcome to de Woude. I'll show you to your room."

A rooster's crow woke me before dawn. After rubbing the sleep out of my eyes and splashing water on my face, I threw on my clothes. Then, not even stopping for breakfast, I rode my bike past the church on a street called Woude to the northeastern end of the village, stopping in front of a large farm. I smirked. The people in this place seemed short on imagination; the sign proclaimed that it was called "The Big Farm."

Leaning my bike against the fence, I looked for the doorbell before knocking on the bright orange door. The top panel of the door swung open, revealing a plump blond lady with a baby girl in her arms and a toddler clinging to her skirt.

"Ah, you must be Frits," she said while unlatching the bottom half of the door. "I'm Mevrouw de Boer, and this guy is Steefje."

I smiled at the tow-headed boy and held out my hand, thinking he might like to shake it. Steefje quickly slipped behind his mother, whose eyes crinkled at the corners.

"Yes, well, and this little lady is Elsje."

I touched the baby's soft cheek, trying not to think of another baby who was no more. "You have beautiful children."

"*Bedankt*. Come in," she invited. "Let me show you where you'll be sleeping."

I followed Mevrouw de Boer up the stairs and then up another flight to the attic, which was filled with wonderfully aromatic hay. Better that than mice. In the corner was a cot made up with sheets and a blanket.

"Oh, this looks lovely." I put my *koffer* down.

"It's what we have." Mevrouw de Boer shrugged. "When you're ready, come down to have some breakfast with us. Then Meneer de Boer will show you around the farm."

I didn't need to be invited twice. Already on the way up, the scent of freshly baked bread and the sight of home-churned yellow butter and various homemade jams made my mouth water. I was going to go home weighing double!

After breakfast, Meneer de Boer took over. Adjusting his flat cap before donning his wooden shoes, the farmer led the way. "Well,

Frits, this'll be an education for a city boy like you. You'll have to clean the chicken coops. *Jawel*, you'll be learning a lot!"

"No problem. I helped my brother do that at the boarding school in Den Haag."

He raised his eyebrows. "*Jawel?* In Den Haag? Well, how are you at repairing stuff? You'll have to fix fences."

"Pretty good, I think. I make all kinds of things: radios, plugs, locks, and more. Also, I had to do all the repairs at the children's home in Driebergen, where I lived during the war."

"Well, this'll be a new one." Meneer de Boer's blue eyes twinkled. "You'll have to take the bull to visit the cows on a regular basis."

Losing some of my bravado, I stopped mid-stride. "Sir?"

"*Jawel.* Just load him into my rowboat and take him on down the canal to my field. When he's finished doing his business, bring him home to sleep it off."

I searched the man's face carefully. Was he joking? "Um, the rowboat seems rather…um…small. Will a bull fit?"

Meneer de Boer's eyes crinkled at the corners. "*Jawel.*"

"And is it safe?" I squeaked.

"*Jawel!*" he cackled. "You see, on the way there, he knows where you're taking him, and he's delighted to go. On the way back, he's as mellow as you'd expect."

I quickly covered my cheeks with my hands so my employer wouldn't see them turn red, but it was too late.

This turned out to be my favorite task. The bull was amazingly cooperative, and while he was busy, I gave him some privacy by lying in the soft green grass and watching the clouds go by.

Mostly, my stay in de Woude was idyllic. Once the farm work was complete, my time was my own. I could ride my ancient bicycle around town, enjoy the profusion of flowers on every street, watch children play, and chat with locals. That is, until the thunderstorm.

Late one afternoon, the sky grew dark with clouds. The wind pushed me down the street, and I was glad to slam the door in its face when I got back to the farmhouse. Meneer de Boer met me in the front hall.

"Oi, Frits. I'm glad you made it back before the rain began."

I eyed the raincoats he and his wife were wearing. "Are you going out?"

"*Jawel.* We're having dinner at the small farm. Can you watch *de kindertjes*?"

"There's pea soup ready on the stove, and I made fresh bread today," added Mevrouw de Boer.

I eyed Steefje, who already had his arms wrapped around my leg, and his drooling sister, Elsje. "Sure!"

Mevrouw de Boer passed Elsje to me before bending down to kiss Steefje, whose thumb drifted into his mouth. "Be good, Steefje! I'll check on you when I get home, and you'll see me in the morning."

The evening went as well as could be expected. At least some of the soup went in their mouths and they either wore or painted with the rest. Finally, having bathed, put the children to bed, and cleaned the table, chairs, and floor, I sank into a chair by the front window. I planned to read the book on how to repair farm machinery that my employer lent me.

By now, the wind was howling, whipping leaves off the trees, and the peals of thunder were deafening. I lifted my head to listen for cries but heard nothing. It seemed the children were sleeping soundly. Just then, lightning lit the sky, so I got to my feet to watch the show nature was offering.

In only a matter of minutes, the scent of smoke tickled my nostrils. I'd been careful to turn the stove off, so what was the source? Better check on the children. They were still sleeping, but the smell in their room was even more pungent. I left the room and looked up. Was that a curl of smoke coming from under my bedroom door? I climbed the next flight of stairs, carefully opened the door, and jumped back in shock. The thatched roof and the dry hay right under it were on fire.

I grabbed a blanket from my bed and raced down the stairs toward the children's room. A piece of burning timber from the roof hit me in the back but only caused a momentary delay as I gasped in pain. Steefje and Elsje were fast asleep, but I grabbed them out of their beds, tucking one under each arm. I ran down the next flight of stairs as if wolves were after me. Once in the front garden, I wrapped the now-crying children in the blanket, sheltering them as best I could with my body.

The rain was still pelting down but the sky was alight with fire and smoke. In no time, most of the villagers joined me in watching the big farm burn to the ground. When the de Boers arrived, breathless and wild-eyed, little was left of their home. Snatching their children, they peppered them with kisses, sobbing out their gratitude to me.

The family and I were given rooms above the restaurant. I lay on my stomach all night, biting my lips against the pain, but so thankful that the children were safe. It was only the next day that I sought medical attention.

Unfortunately, since the farmhouse was gone, there wasn't work for me. Once my burns made it possible to travel, I returned to my tiny room in Den Haag. This meant I had less money to give Moeder, but at least I had time to study and prepare for my final year at the NUTS school. Perhaps I could graduate early.

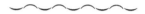

Dear Frits,

You'll never guess what I'm going to be. The bad news is that the after-primary-school test at Wassenaar confirmed I can't read very well. I knew that! The good news is that I know what a fat skimmer is. So, I'm training as a cook and waiter. Mama is once again rid of me.

The school is Catholic; I'm learning to say the "Our Father" and "Hail Mary," among other things. If we open our eyes while praying, the teacher shouts, "God d*mn, close your eyes," right in the middle of the prayer. It almost makes me want to open them!

Wow! God burned down a farm because of you? You must have done more than had your eyes open.

Your better-looking brother, Jan

I slowly lowered my brother's letter. Yes, he was quiet around most people, but with me, he sparkled. I missed him, especially now, while Henk was on vacation with his parents, and I was living a solitary existence in my room.

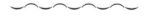

1950 After tucking my satchel, complete with my precious slide rule, compass, and protractor, into the luggage carrier at the back of my bike, I swung my leg over the saddle. I should study. But the sun was shining, and the breeze was tickling my nose with scents of Fall. Schoolwork could wait. "Hey Guys, let's go to the sand dunes."

I glanced over my shoulder at my group of friends. Of late, Ellie, a blue-eyed angel with blond ringlets, had caught my eye. Would she be coming? Of course, it would appear too desperate actually to stop and see, so I cycled on in the lead.

"Frits, slow down."

I stopped immediately upon hearing her sweet tones. My heart beat just a bit faster.

"Oh, hi; I wondered if you'd be able to make it." I crossed my ankles and leaned on my bike in a laidback fashion, only to have my cover blown when it and I fell over.

Ellie giggled. "Yes, but I can't stay for long. Mamma expects me to help with dinner."

I nodded as if I understood. "I guess you have to help a lot with so many children in your family, right?"

"Eight kids do eat a lot of food! How many children are there in your family?"

"Um, there's just the two of us. I have a younger brother. Oh, look at that kite!" Changing the subject away from my living situation seemed wise. Few in my circle knew I lived in a rented room. I might like this girl, but there was no way I was about to let her into my secret pain.

"The beach is full of them today. But, about your family, aren't they Catholic? Why so few children?"

I shifted uncomfortably. It seemed she wasn't going to let this line of questioning go. "We lost my father during the war," I mumbled. "Let's go."

Ellie's eyes were filled with compassion but quickly became curiously blank. "Oh, sure, sure. I'll race you!"

That was the last time Ellie joined our group. Henk told me someone informed her that I wasn't Catholic. Worse, because I didn't elaborate on my father, she suspected he died because he was Jewish. Her parents absolutely forbade her from spending time with people like me! The end of the war did not usher in the end of prejudice.

Frits, Jan, and Poemel, on Moeder's balcony, 1948. (top)

Frits's report card, 1949/50. (bottom)

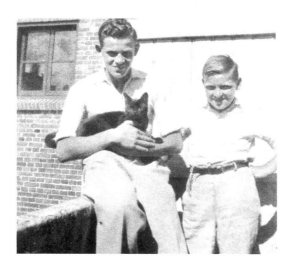

Moeder and Vader, 1950.

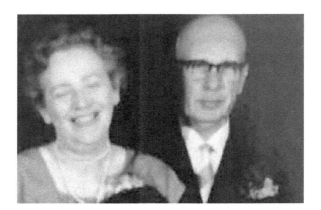

10

THE DREAM

I was done! With high school, that is. The round of exams administered by the government was thorough, to say the least. We first took the B exams, which selected students with superior abilities in mathematics and science. Next came the A essay tests, which were more general in nature. Finally, all students took oral exams at de Malieveld in Den Haag. I figured the ultimate goal was to drain our brains of all that the past years had squashed into them.

Now, a group of chattering youngsters gathered around the board where our results would soon be posted. Despite only being 17, I was hoping I'd passed and would graduate from the NUTS school. Perhaps they would even deem me qualified to go on in science.

Standing in the crowd, my hands started twirling. My chest ached. Had I done enough? I'd studied every minute I could, but it wasn't easy while existing with no heat and very little food. I grinned briefly, remembering what Henk wrote in my school book: "Evenblij will have to work a bit harder. Otherwise, he will most gloriously fail."

But I didn't just want to pass. I wanted so much more: marks high enough to allow me entrance into the Middelbare Technische School (MTS, a polytechnic school). There, I could train to be an electrical engineer. That would be my dream come true.

The government official parted our anxious company like Moses parted the Red Sea and strode through to tack the exam results to the board. We flowed back to stand in front of it, our eyes anxiously moving down the column of names to our own. Henk's were faster than mine.

"Evenblij, you dog! Your B exam results are incredible. You came out top of the class in math and physics!"

"Let me see!" I shoved him out of my way. He was right—and my marks in the A exam subjects weren't too bad either. Well, most of them, anyway.

What about Henk? I scanned until I reached his last name. "First in foreign languages! What? Are you planning on being a diplomat? Or maybe a spy! You could talk via your ham radio!"

Henk punched me in the arm. "Wow, Evenblij, you really stunk at some things! Your marks in German and Esperanto are atrocious. Guess you won't be a spy."

"*Nee,* I'll just invent a better ham radio for you to use. Or maybe a code… We could work together."

We strolled away from the board and threw ourselves down on the grass. Henk stuck a blade in his mouth before asking, "What are your plans for the summer?"

"I'm going back to de Woude to work. Since the big farm burned down, I'll be at another farm. I did like it there. What about you?"

Henk grimaced. "Helping my parents in the shop, as usual. What about in September?"

I snapped my fingers. "That's right! I forgot to tell you. I heard from MTS. They said I would have a place if my exam results were good. And they are! Now, I'm on my way…to becoming an electrical engineer."

"Wha…you were accepted?" Henk raised himself on an elbow to stare at me. "Congratulations! That's wonderful!"

"*Bedankt.*" It was a significant accomplishment, but somehow, Papa not seeing it diminished my joy. But only a little. Moeder, of course, wouldn't care. I deflected further questions. "What're you going to do after the summer?"

Henk sat up and put his arms around his legs. "I'm not sure. Although it would be fun to do further schooling, my family needs me to help…"

I clapped my friend on the back. A show of sympathy would be unmanly, but distraction might work.

"Well, let's see if it's sunny tomorrow. If you can beat me in a race around the pier, I'll write you an MTS certificate for your bedroom wall myself."

"Ha! I could win that race with my hands tied behind my back."

"We'll see. As long as it's not freezing cold, meet me there at 11 sharp."

I could see the sun shining through my window in the morning, even with the curtains closed. No school. No work yet. I was free and going to meet Henk for a race. I couldn't wipe the grin from my face.

Pulling my ham radio equipment from under the bed, I tuned in to Henk. "*Goedemorgen*, lazy bones. You better have a nutritious breakfast because I'm putting on my racing gear."

A bit of static, and then Henk's response came through. "11 am. Be there."

After pulling on my clothes, I sat down to my favorite breakfast: boiled eggs. In this case, eggs that I'd boiled a couple of days before. Thus fortified, I jumped on my bike and made for the pier.

The beach was full of holiday-makers, tourists, and even residents of Scheveningen enjoying the relatively rare sunshine.

Henk, always one to enjoy attention, strode up, shouting, "Ah, so here's the man who will lose the race. Everyone, meet Frits Evenblij."

I bowed theatrically to the little crowd who stopped to watch us. "Oh, my friend, you're wrong. So wrong. I'm going to win." I whipped off my shirt and flexed my muscles, causing a few girls to titter.

We had now drawn more onlookers, so Henk continued the fun, taking off his pants and twirling them around his head. A few older ladies gasped, but they kept watching. After all, what might these wild young men do next?

"Come on, loser, time to prove what you're saying." I placed my clothing and shoes in a pile and crouched in the starting pose. Henk joined me.

"Ready, set, go!" called someone in the crowd.

We both set off swimming with powerful strokes. The icy, exhilarating water of the North Sea only sped us up. First, Henk was in the lead, and then I was. We rounded the head of the pier, and on the home stretch, Henk swam by me. By now, my chest hurt, but I powered through, once again passing Henk. I felt sand under my knees and realized I'd won! But only by a fingernail.

Many members of the original crowd had followed the race and were now cheering for us both. Henk stood up and threw me a seashell. "Here's the winner's prize!" he crowed.

Unfortunately, while I was an excellent swimmer, I'd never learned to catch. It fell to the ground. Henk chuckled. "Guess he doesn't want it."

The following week, after a quick stop at home to see Jan, I cycled to de Woude. Rebuilding the big farm was still a work in progress, but the farmer had given me a good reference. I had a job at the small farm right across the street.

My eyes crinkled at the corners, seeing the little ferry with its wizened old driver approaching. "Hoi Frits, back again?"

"Of course. Where else could a person find an outdoor job in such a beautiful place?"

The wrinkled man puffed up his chest and grinned widely. "It's the best place in the world. I should know. I was born here. And did I tell you I used to be a sailor? I've been almost everywhere!"

I chuckled. "That's amazing. I hope one day I'll have the chance to visit other countries. Meanwhile, I'll enjoy de Woude. At least, I know it has the best storms."

Little did I know my words would prove prophetic. Only a month later, lightning hit the little farm, and it burned to the ground. Fortunately, we all escaped unscathed, but I was once again without employment. And the fire destroyed my old bicycle. No villager would house me, so I stayed in the inn until I could leave.

The next week, I strapped my *koffer* onto the luggage carrier of my new bicycle. The villagers had banded together to buy it for me. To my surprise, most of them followed me to the ferry. How kind to see me off! I turned to wave, only to hear someone shout, "And don't come back!"

I shrugged. I knew there were more beautiful places in the world and meant to see them. Silly superstitious people!

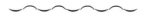

Despite this meaning a significant financial hit, I was kind of happy about being unable to work. It meant I could begin preparing for MTS. A degree in engineering would be a dream come true, and I meant to do all I could to gain one.

I looked around my tiny room. Of course, while in college, I would still have to depend on Moeder for help with rent. But I hoped that eventually, I would have a lucrative career: then neither she nor anyone else would have power over my life. September couldn't come soon enough.

When I first entered the MTS lecture hall, the bright sun could not hold a candle to my joy. Imagine! I would indulge my lifelong fascination with electricity, physics, and mathematics every day, all day. My cheeks hurt from a smile that persisted even while I took careful notes on everything the teacher said. Since I couldn't afford textbooks, I was determined to get as much information as possible from class. I hoped the books would be available in the library.

As soon as the lecture ended, I tucked my precious notebook into my bag and began jogging to the next class.

"Hey, wait!"

Glancing over my shoulder, I saw a dark-haired string bean of a man smiling at me. "Yeah?"

"I saw you in class. You sure were taking good notes. What's your name? Want to be study partners?"

A furrow appeared between my brows. "Um, my name is Frits. With an *s*, of course. Who are you?"

"Oops, sorry. I'm Arie, your new best friend."

I grinned. This man reminded me of Trouble. Of course, I was too old to get into the same scrapes, but a friend in this place would be welcome. "Good to meet you, Arie, my new best friend."

Arie looped his arm through mine. "And what do I see there? The Disciplinary Regulations?"

Before I could stop him, Arie pulled the paper I was clutching out of my hand. This document had been passed out to all newcomers, and, in one of my less guarded moments, I'd "altered" some of the wording. For example, I changed "Talking, whistling, humming, and walking around are not tolerated" to "Talking, whistling, humming, and walking around are highly appreciated." I didn't like people ordering me around, not even on paper.

Arie's guffaws as he read attracted the attention of other students, but I was relieved he didn't show the document to them before returning it to me. "You'd better hide this, Frits with an *s*!"

I quickly stuffed the paper into my bag, arranging my features into a picture of innocence. "I have no idea what you're referring to, sir."

"Come on, you mighty peculiar man. After our next class and lunch, I'll show you a good place for studying."

Our minds and stomachs satisfied, we sat down in a secluded part of the college library, and soon, both of us were lost, immersed in the wonders of electricity. Every weekday, I learned more and more about my favorite subject. Every evening and weekend, I worked on problems and figured out how to wire things so they run better—Frits heaven.

"Oh, my goodness, are you studying again?" Arie's eyes bugged out when he rounded the corner and spotted me seated in my favorite place in the library, surrounded by papers and books. "All work and no play…come with me. You should join a fraternity. If nothing else, the connections will help you in your future career."

I stood and stretched to get the kinks out of my neck and back before carefully putting my precious papers away. I'd actually been figuring out an anagram, but Arie didn't need to know that. "Sure, I can spare an hour or two."

So it was that on October 14, 1950, I was inducted into an MTS fraternity, a brotherhood of people just like me. Like me in terms of their passion for electrical engineering, anyway. None of them had any idea about my past, and I saw no reason to enlighten them. After all, I was on my way to a bright new future! And I knew Papa would've been proud.

Entrance certificate for MTS, 1950. (top)
Frits studying for MTS, 1950. (bottom)

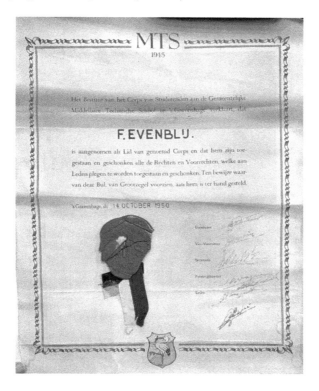

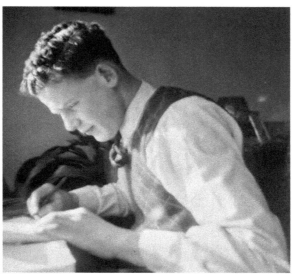

The MTS instructions for behavior that Frits 'doctored,' 1950.

—

MIDDELBARE TECHNISCHE SCHOOL (Gem.)
Sneeuwbalstraat 137   Tel. 390659   's-Gravenhage

DISCIPLINAIRE VOORSCHRIFTEN.

Iedere leerling zal straks in zijn loopbaan ondervinden,
dat in alle technische bureaux en tekenkamers absolute stilte
~~vereist~~ is. Dat is noodzakelijk ten einde andere niet te hin-
deren en productief te kunnen werken. Gepraat, gefluit, neuriën,
en rondlopen wordt daar ~~niet getolereerd~~. Maak deze gedragslijn
reeds op school tot een gewoonte.

In verband met het bovenstaande wordt tijdens de tekenlessen:
praten, fluiten, neuriën en rondlopen ten strengste verboden. na te laten
Iedereen moet gedurende de gehele les op zijn plaats blijven en zingen en
absolute stilte in acht ~~nemen~~. Het ~~lenen~~ van tekengereedschappen,
papier of boeken wordt niet geaccepteerd. Iedereen moet daarom
van alles, wat hij voor zijn werk nodig heeft, voorzien zijn.

~~Het niet~~ na komen van al deze voorschriften zal leiden tot ver-
wijdering uit de tekenzaal. Wordt iemand voor de derde maal ver-
wijderd, dan volgt voor hem een schorsing met alle daaraan ver-
bonden ~~nadelige~~ gevolgen voor zijn ~~studie~~. meisje

Hinder een ander ~~niet~~ en breng U zelf niet in moeilijkheden!
's Morgens en 's middags vóór ~~de aanvang~~ het begin der lessen gaan er twee
belsignalen.

Tussen beide signalen verlopen enkele ~~minuten~~ uren, vóór het
eerste belsignaal moet door ~~~~ daartoe aangewezen leerlingen
de tekenbanken ~~in het lokaal~~ worden gebracht, vóór het ~~tweede~~ derde belsignaal dient elke leerling voor zijn tekenbord ~~~~ opgespannen
~~tekening~~ te staan.

Vijf minuten vóór het einde der lessen moet begonnen worden
met het opbergen van tekengereedschap e.d. uren
Enkele ~~minuten~~ vóór het einde ~~der lessen~~ van het jaar brengen t de ~~beide~~
~~boven genoemde~~ leerlingen ~~~~ met tekeningen ~~weer~~ achter op de fiets
~~daartoe bestemde plaats~~. naar huis.

ik en De Baas

182

11

THE CHANGE

1951 Spring rain pelted my head and streamed down my neck as I rode, making the journey much more arduous than it might have been. I wasn't looking forward to spending time with Moeder, but wanted to catch up with Jan, who would also be there. I grinned, imagining him in an apron and chef's hat.

It was after dark when I arrived at the house, shook the water out of my clothing, and pressed the bell, just like I wasn't part of the family. The door swung open with a creak, and the lighted doorway framed Vader. Clothed in brown dress pants, a blue shirt, a tie, and a matching vest, he came forward and solemnly offered me his hand. "*Goedenavond*, Frits."

I leaned my bike against the wall and wiped my hands on my pants before formally shaking his hand. "*Goedenavond*, Vader."

His touch made my hair stand on end, but I showed no discomfort. Tolerating Vader was a prerequisite for seeing my brother.

"Come in," he intoned. "Your mother is in the living room."

I suppressed a wry smile as I went through to the elegantly appointed living quarters. Of course, she was. Moeder was in her happy place, seated on the chaise lounge beside a side table sporting a crystal glass of red wine and a small bowl of nuts. Both were set on what looked like a silver platter. Poemel was curled up at her feet.

Moeder languidly stretched a hand toward me after carefully adjusting her woolen skirt around her silken hose. "Ah, Frits. Forgive me for not getting up. You're much later than we expected, and I'm so exhausted."

I glanced past her out the window to where the rain still fell thick and fast. "I'm sorry, Moeder. It's hard to cycle in this kind of weather."

Vader cleared his throat before Moeder responded with a plastic smile. "Always complaining, aren't you? Well, I'm afraid we didn't save you any dinner. You could perhaps make yourself *een boterham*."

I suppressed a sigh and forcefully stopped my shoulders from rounding around my empty stomach. Why did my heart still lodge this tiny, but fervent, kernel of hope that Moeder would show me love? "I'm not hungry. *Bedankt*."

"Good. Vader and I want to discuss something with you, and it's better done in person."

I quickly sank into Papa's chair. This sounded serious. "Tell me, Moeder."

After exchanging a glance with Vader, Moeder continued. "I wish you would stop with this ridiculous *moeder* business."

I remained silent, schooling my features to give no indication that I'd even heard her.

Moeder drew in a deep breath before launching in. "The landlord where you're staying on the Barentszstraat has raised the rent. You'll have to move out."

Relief flooded me. Why was this such a big deal? "Okay, I'll find another room. A cheaper one. That shouldn't be a problem." I got to my feet to go and find Jan.

Moeder held up her hand. "Sit. I haven't finished. Vader and I have decided that, since you're now 18, it's no longer appropriate for us to pay your rent."

Dumbfounded, my brain went into overdrive. "Umm, I'm in the middle of college. MTS has a rule that I can't have a job. So…can I live here?"

Moeder tittered. "*Nee, nee,* of course not! You couldn't afford what we'd charge. *Nee,* you'll have to quit the MTS and get a full-time job."

Quit? My dream? I closed my eyes, and my fingers tightened on the armrests that still bore the imprint of Papa's hands.

"Frits! Are you listening to me?"

The loud buzzing in my ears had drowned her out. "What d…d…did you say?" My voice shook.

Moeder huffed impatiently. "Stop with the dramatics! You're an adult--old enough to be responsible. We're actually prepared to be very generous, since your job probably won't cover the rent. We've discussed it, and if you send us everything you earn, we'll help by paying the entire bill. Of course, we'll expect you to pay us back eventually."

My face alternately grew pale and flushed as my heart struggled to beat, not that Moeder noticed. I'd fervently hoped that she would be proud of what I was achieving and want to support me in it. Evidently not. I'd need to appeal to what *was* important to her: prestige.

After taking a deep breath, I leaned forward, ignoring the tears streaming down my face. "Moeder, think about it! I passed the NUTS school with top grades. That means I'll probably do well at the MTS. And, if I finish the electrical engineering course, I'll be able to earn so much more than I could now."

Moeder opened her mouth to interrupt, but I pressed on. "You might even be able to move to a bigger apartment in a better neighborhood. And buy more silver trays!"

"Oh, this?" Moeder touched the tray where her wine sat. "It's not silver; it's just a bauble Jan picked up for me. Regardless, Vader and I have discussed this extensively. Our minds are made up. You'll turn in your resignation to MTS and start looking for a job immediately. And I hope you're grateful for all we've done for you until now." She picked up the book on her lap, effectively closing the discussion.

I leaped to my feet, causing Vader to move quickly to stand beside Moeder. Did he imagine I'd hit her? And, if I was so inclined, did the old man actually think he could fight me off, a young man who spent his free time bicycling, swimming, and otherwise being active? I rolled my eyes and smirked at him before turning to Moeder with fists clenched and eyes blazing.

"You..you…you've never done anything but reject me and try to ruin my life—well, now you've accomplished your goal." Poemel jumped off the chaise lounge and hid, but I continued shouting. "C…c…congratulations! *Ja*, you'll have my measly income, but you just lost yourself a son. I despise you! You are nothing to me! You might not care now, but think about when you're old, and Vader is gone. Remember my words! I'll never forgive you. Never!"

Drawn into the room by my raised voice, Jan stood wide-eyed, his mouth hanging open. I roughly pushed past him before slamming the door on my way out. It was finished. Utterly finished.

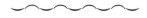

The trouble was there were few places in Den Haag where a person could sit throughout a windy, wet night. I'd forgotten my bicycle in my haste, so stumbled through the streets aimlessly until I ended at the railroad station. Shivering while watching the hands of the clock move to midnight, then 1 am, then 2 am, 3, 4…, I sat throughout that long night, chewing on my sorry life and how it was all her fault.

Moving from the Congo and away from the boys—Moeder's fault because she didn't like the weather. Living in Driebergen, where we were physically abused and emotionally neglected—Moeder's fault since she didn't want to dirty her lily-white hands with being a mother. Papa's death—Moeder's fault because she'd been on vacation instead of caring for him as a wife should. Tante Esther, Oom Henri, and my cousins being taken to Auschwitz—maybe Moeder's fault, since her father was Jewish, she never wore a yellow star, and I now knew she hated her brother. Concordia College—Moeder's fault because she never wanted Jan and me and was too desperate to get rid of us to thoroughly vet the places we were sent. Deep down, I knew some of these accusations made little sense, but was far beyond caring.

Furiously wiping my tears with one hand while rubbing my aching chest with the other, my heart filled up with rage. I hated Moeder with a passion. She'd taken away everything good in my life. I had nothing left at all.

I needn't have bothered working so hard at the NUTS school. I needn't have studied for hours and hours during my two semesters at the MTS. I should never have allowed myself to dream. I'd never be an electrical engineer. I'd never even have a degree.

I rested my chin on my hand as I fumed. I'd probably end up cleaning for my profession! Or cooking, like poor old Jan. I'd never earn enough to make a living, so I was doomed to be in her power forever, the old witch yanking my chain and dictating my life.

I already suspected I'd never have Moeder's love, but this was worse. If she had her way, I'd never be free of her. I figured the only way out was death, but wasn't entirely sure suicide was a good idea. After all, then she'd win. She'd probably dance on my grave. Well, if she remembered where it was.

"Hey you, the station is closed. Move on," a watchman ordered.

Typical! I wasn't even welcome here, where hobos spend their time. Loudly exhaling, I clambered stiffly to my feet. Where could I go? There was nowhere, so I wandered the dark, wet streets until morning. At sunrise, bells started ringing all over the city. It was Sunday.

I could go into a church. Today, their doors would be open, and at least it'd be dry, if not warm. Following the worshippers into the sanctuary of a Catholic church, I hung my head, well aware that I looked pretty rough. My clothing was soaked; I hadn't shaved; my face was tear-stained; I was shaking from cold; and my shoes squelched and squirted water with every step.

An older woman's touch on my elbow gave me a start. "Here, young man, sit next to me."

Her warm brown eyes and wrinkled cheeks were wreathed with a friendly smile. I gingerly took the seat she offered, ensuring that my wet clothing didn't come into contact with her brown and gray checked woolen coat.

Paying me no heed, the lady rummaged in her oversized bag and pulled out a warm *stroopwafel*.

I frowned and quickly looked away. Surely churches don't allow eating! But she did seem like a sweet, older woman, so maybe they'd make an allowance for her.

"I guess I knew you'd be here," she whispered, turning my trembling hand over with her wizened paw before giving me the treat. "Or maybe I heard your stomach growling. I just wish I brought more than one!"

I amended my thoughts as I whispered my thanks. A sweet, *weird*, old woman. No matter. I gratefully accepted her offering, taking mouth-watering bites when nobody was looking. Fortunately, we were at the back, where the poor people sit.

"Here," she murmured, placing her coat over my lap. "You need this more than I do."

Gradually, my shivering ceased. The priest droned on, and I luxuriated in the warmth of my new friend's coat. Exhausted from being in extremis all night, my eyes grew heavy, and I fell fast asleep. In my dreams, I traveled back several years to a different church service in another place. I was desperately miserable then, too, having just lost my cousins and Keetie. Even in sleep, my fists clenched as I again heard the minister say that forgiveness is essential.

A particularly loud word from the pulpit woke me, but because the priest was speaking Latin, I tuned him out. Instead, I revisited the sermon that I'd heard so long ago. It was still strangely fresh in my mind, and I clearly remembered something I'd meditated on ever since: the pastor in Driebergen's claim that forgiveness benefits the one who forgives more than the one who is forgiven. I still had my doubts, but I recalled that he compared anger to poison, which damages the angry person. I was sure that my rage against Moeder was justified, but my roiling stomach and aching chest suggested that I was indeed drinking poison.

My eyebrows drew together. I definitely didn't want Moeder to get away with anything! But was this the way? Would holding this grudge ensure she suffered? In my mind's eyes, I again saw her coolly picking up her book, even while the tears streamed from my eyes. It was painfully evident that she neither knew nor cared about the hurt she caused. So why bother getting upset?

Yes, her treatment of her sons was beyond horrible. That was indisputable. But I remembered the pastor addressing that issue, as well. "Forgiveness is only necessary if an offense has indeed occurred." In other words, forgiveness in no way diminishes the gravity of the offense. But, like cutting an electrical wire, it short-circuits the damage by breaking the tie between the offender and victim.

So much of what had happened in my life was unforgivable. The actions of Zuster Dermout in beating me and locking me in the attic definitely were. All the atrocities of WWII were absolutely unforgivable. Honestly, even God allowing my beloved and much-needed Papa to die was, in my eyes, unforgivable. Yup. I was furious with Moeder, Zuster Dermout, the Nazis, and God. All of them.

But now I started to see that I needed to be free from my rage if I were to survive and eventually overcome my past. I had to stop drinking poison, and those ties of anger had to be broken. With a quick nod, I made my decision. I would forgive—well, except for the Nazis, of course. That would be a step too far. And, as much as I could for everyone else, I would forget. Would I trust Moeder again? No. Would I expect her to change? Of course not. Would it work? Who knows?

I vaguely remembered the pastor talking about dusting off our feet against those who offend us. That's what I would do: just move on.

Now, should I pray? Early in my life, the wonders of the universe convinced me that some kind of god exists. Experience led me to believe He's as interested in us as a dog is in its fleas. But what if I was wrong? I shrugged and decided to hedge my bets by praying. At least, the action would solidify my personal vow.

Feeling silly, I closed my eyes and, for the first time in my life, really talked to God. "*Goedemiddag* Great Intelligence, this is Frits here. I don't know if You listen to people, but just in case, I need Your help. For the rest of my life, I want to forgive and forget. I guess I'll do it, even if you're not listening or don't exist because it makes sense. So, for now, Amen."

Then, just in case He was holding my past behavior against me, I whispered the last verse of my favorite hymn. "Whatever the future may bring, the Lord's hand is leading me. I believe the Savior's promise, life with him eternally."

Transaction accomplished; I raised my chin to face the future. I would work toward carving out my own life and be satisfied with that. Maybe then Moeder would be proud of me. Glancing around, I raised my eyebrows in surprise. Somehow, while I'd been thinking and praying, the service had finished. My elderly companion was gone, as was her coat. Had she even been real? I checked my lap for *stroopwafel* crumbs and brushed them onto the floor.

Not yet ready to see Vader and Moeder, I ambled toward Henk's house, still deep in thought. What would forgiving mean? The key seemed to be in not exacting revenge—not damaging the body, emotions, wallet, or reputation of the ones who'd hurt me. I'd never had any intention of beating someone up, but was it possible that my shouting at Moeder hurt her feelings? If so, could I stop? Maybe. Probably not.

For me, a pretty unimportant and ineffective youth, the best I figured I could do was to refrain from gossip--not to talk about those who'd harmed me. If I could do this, I might eventually forget what they did. I hoped that God, if He exists, would understand I was trying the best I could. Maybe He would even help.

I spotted the warm light shining through the windows of Henk's home just as the rain stopped. His parents welcomed me as if I were their own, no questions asked, and I spent a few blissful days with the family. Watching Henk interact with them filled my heart with longing; I attempted to quell envy. It wouldn't help, and from now on, I intended only to do and feel what would bring me closer to my goal.

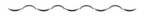

Early in June, I stopped by Vader and Moeder's house. Moeder, who showed no relief at my reappearance, was on her chaise lounge, a cup of tea, a piece of cake, and a tiny fork beside her.

My stomach churned, but I forced the words out anyway. "Moeder, I'm here to apologize. I'm sorry I got so angry about having to work."

"Finally, you see reason! Why are you always so difficult?" Moeder took a bite and carefully wiped her lips before continuing. "Now, are you ready to do as you're told?"

I took a deep breath. "Yes, I already resigned from the MTS, but need somewhere to live. Can I stay here?"

Moeder shook her head. *"Nee,* that won't work, but you're in luck. I found you a place with Meneer and Mevrouw Verbeek, friends of mine whose son is a colonel in the army. They want to earn a bit of money by filling his room. I'll pay your rent there until you find a job. Of course, once you do, when you earn enough, you'll need to cover your rent, as well as give me a bit of money that will go towards paying me back."

My nails bit into my palms. "Yes, Moeder. *Dank u wel*, Moeder. What's the address?"

"The van Hoornbeekstraat 73. They're expecting you."

I turned and left before I said more.

To my surprise, the Verbeeks were a very kindhearted couple, and I immediately warmed to them. They showed me to a third-floor room, which was furnished with a freshly made-up bed, a small dresser, and a bookcase. There was even a rug on the floor.

I unpacked my *koffer* and began walking the streets searching for work. Here at least my good grades at MTS came in useful. I was almost immediately offered a position with the Vereenigde Accountants Kantooren (VAK) in Den Haag, starting on July 1. It wasn't engineering, but my job would involve mathematics.

Every weekday, I rode my bicycle to work, put in a full day, rode to my room, and studied. I hoped that, if I worked hard, I could eventually return to the MTS. I gazed at the budget I made. Out of the 300 guilders I earned every month (about $160), I had to pay $54 in rent and give $26 to Moeder. Food, clothing, incidentals, and savings were to come out of the remaining $80, but who needs clothes?

Whenever I felt stirrings of anger about my circumstances or exasperation with Moeder, I remembered my vow to forgive and forget. If I didn't forget, at least I mostly managed to distract myself and stuff the pain down deep. Surely God, if He were as loving as the pastor suggested, would understand that I was doing the best I could. If He existed, that is. And, slowly, slowly, as the anger was pushed out of my heart, the space left for love grew.

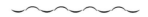

1952 One aspect of working at the VAK was that, apart from studying, I had my weekends free. Too free. My MTS friends were occupied with classes and homework, and I'd lost touch with all except Arie. I couldn't handle seeing them anyway, knowing I'd had to leave. Henk had to work in his parents' shop on Saturdays and help with his siblings on Sundays. Jan was cooking. Although I enjoyed the nearby Scheveningse bosjes and the beach and loved playing with electronics, I needed another outlet.

After Moeder overheard me discussing the problem with Jan, she advised me to enroll for lessons at the Anne and Wim Smidt School for dance in Scheveningen. She thought it would be a good way for me to meet a suitable girl. I just thought it might be fun—a diversion.

On the first day of class, February 3, I hesitantly entered the dance studio, smoothing down my curly mop and straightening the only clothing I had. The shirt was threadbare and the pants were a little short in the leg, but at least they were clean.

"Good to see you, Meneer Evenblij. Your mother told me to expect you, and I'm so glad you came." Mevrouw Smidt, a distant relation, glided in my direction before holding out her hand. "I've partnered you with one of our newest teachers." She stopped to wink and continued under her breath, "She's also the prettiest one."

I rolled my eyes. She'd clearly received the matchmaker memo from Moeder. Then, I saw her. My mouth went dry—she was quite the most beautiful girl I'd ever laid eyes upon. Her wavy brown hair, sapphire eyes, hourglass figure, and graceful movements would have been enough to leave me speechless, but her smile was the clincher. It lit up the entire room.

"Meneer Frits Evenblij, this is Juffrouw Meta Bisschop. But we're pretty informal here, so feel free to address each other by your first names." Mevrouw Smidt drifted away, not that I noticed.

Meta tilted her head to meet my eyes and offered her hand. "Pleased to meet you, Frits. I'll be teaching you to dance."

"Um, uh…" I pressed my lips together to stop myself from making any other brilliant noises.

"We'll begin with the foxtrot. Let's start without music, shall we?" My dream-come-true pointed to the dance floor.

Still dumbstruck, I nodded and followed her, feeling like a galumphing bear.

Meta's eyes crinkled, and she reeled off a list of instructions. Her voice was so low-pitched and melodic that it was hard to focus on what she was saying. I was mesmerized.

"Are you listening?" With her hands on her hips, Meta pierced me with her eyes.

I dug my nails into my palms, cleared my throat, and sucked in a huge breath. I had to say something! "Of course, but c...c...could you repeat what you said so I g...g...get it straight in my mind?"

She complied while demonstrating with her feet. Trying to ignore her slender ankles, I followed her directions. That is until I became aware that she was giggling.

"Frits, your legs aren't made of wood. Try bending your knees a bit."

My face grew hot, and I refocused fiercely, counting under my breath, "1, 2, 3, 4, 1, 2, 3, 4..."

"Ouch!"

I looked up in horror, realizing I'd inadvertently stepped on the angel's toes. "I'm so sorry. I'm n...n...not really a natural d...d...dancer."

Meta grinned while hopping around and rubbing her foot. "I noticed! Don't worry. You'll improve." She exchanged glances with another teacher whose blue eyes were twinkling.

"Who's that?"

"My sister and best friend, Sieglinde. You'll meet her later. Now, let's try it again."

The following week was equally disastrous. "I don't know. I think I'll never get the hang of it," I muttered after stepping on Meta's toes again.

"Oh, don't give up so fast. You just need more practice." She paused while tapping her lip. "I know! We have church dances on Saturday nights. You could come! Sieglinde and I will both be there."

I was more than willing to go, but it soon became painfully apparent that I really didn't fit in. Her church friends were reluctant to accept someone who wasn't Catholic. I wondered how they'd feel if they knew about my Jewish heritage!

Meta had an answer for that—something I was to learn she often did. She, Sieglinde, and a few close friends held dances in her parents' third-floor bedroom, which had a linoleum floor and minimal furniture. As we danced to music coming from the gramophone in the living room on the second floor, I grinned. It was cranked up loud, and I couldn't imagine Moeder putting up with this!

Later, looking around the small but crowded living room of Meta's cozy home at Leeuwardensestraat 1, I beamed like a cat that had fallen into an ocean of cream. This is what I'd always wanted, not the cool elegance of Moeder's aristocratic house. Warmth. Love. Laughter. Even singing. I was so glad that Meta could enjoy it all, especially since I already suspected she might be the one.

The problem was, Meta was very young—barely 17—and while she'd been friendly toward me, that was all. Seeing as she was still in high school, I wondered how to get to know her better. Perhaps, I thought, the indirect route would be best. After all, it gave Meta an easy escape since she probably wouldn't return my interest.

This was the plan: every day after work, I cycled like a madman so I could "happen" to meet Sieglinde after her work at Ougree Exports. And, every day, I graciously accompanied Siegie to her house.

"Frits, you know I already have a boyfriend. So why are you doing this?"

I hung my head and shuffled my feet, feeling my face grow red. "Well, um…"

Sieglinde giggled. "Oh, relax. I'm not an idiot. You want to catch a glimpse of Meta, don't you? I've seen how you look at her."

The hope must have been shining out of my eyes because Sieglinde quickly nodded. "I see. Leave it to me." After that, she consistently invited me to join Meta and her friends whenever they were hanging out.

One day, Sieglinde drew me aside before we reached her home. "I just wanted to warn you. Yesterday, Meta asked me what was going on between you and me. I had to tell her that it wasn't me you were interested in."

I gulped. "And?"

Sieglinde's eyes crinkled at the corners. "Good news. She likes you—a lot. And she was overjoyed once I assured her you aren't as old as she thought."

"Wait! How old did she think I am?"

"Very. Maybe even 25!"

"I'm 18. Maybe it's all this gray hair?" I indicated my curly brown mop with a grin.

Sieglinde shrugged. "I know. Now she knows, too."

I could hardly believe it. Meta returned my interest? Of course, I would have to take it slowly. Because she hadn't even graduated from high school, we only spent time together in the presence of her group of friends. But the walks, parties, and even library visits were blissful for me. I would do anything to be with her. Even dance.

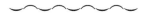

Dear Frits,

I'm sure you know I had a job last summer—in the kitchen of a hotel on the boulevard. Not a bad place, even if the work wasn't my favorite. Mama probably told you. But she for sure didn't tell you I also got an EDUCATION! Such a lot of lovely ladies. Unfortunately, all good things come to an end, and so did the summer.

Now, I'm working as a cook in the restaurant at KLM's (Royal Dutch Airlines) head office. I have to give more than half of what I earn to Mama, so I won't get rich quickly, mainly because I think I may change jobs. Being forced to view KLM President Plesman's dead body gave me a distaste for cooking. Can't imagine why!

Your cooking brother, Jan

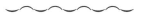

The sun heated my back, and the wind brought scents of heather to my nose, making the bicycle ride to Meta's house a pleasure. I hoped she would be free to go for a walk.

Ringing the bell, I stood first on one foot, then on the other, my hands doing their own peculiar dance of excitement. When the door swung open, I quickly stuffed the offending appendages in my pockets. Would it ever become easy to *doe gewoon*?"

"Oh, hello, Frits," called Meta's father from the top of the steep entrance stairway. "Come on up. I'll see if Meta and Sieglinde are free."

I stifled a wry grin. Meneer Bisschop might be short and balding, but he was fiercely protective of his daughters.

Meta's brother, Ronald, a seven-year-old bundle of energy, accosted me as I mounted the stairs. "Where are you going? Can I come? I'm good at biking. Mama says I'm not allowed to go as far as you do. But maybe if you ask her. I want to see…"

I tousled Ronald's hair. "Maybe another time, Ron."

Meta came out of the kitchen, grinning from ear to ear. My heart stopped at how pretty she looked with her heat-flushed cheeks. She must have been working near the stove.

"Go on into the living room and sit down, Frits." She raised her voice. "Of course, I'd love to go for a walk, and I'm sure Siegie would want to come. But you know how slow she is. She wants to finish the chapter first."

"I'm right here, Meta. I heard Pappa, and I can hear you just fine."

Meta crossed her eyes at Sieglinde, who was curled up in a chair by the *kachel*. "While we wait, how about I make us a picnic?"

I blushed when my stomach let out a loud rumble. With all the exercise I did, I was always hungry.

Meta giggled. "I heard that! I was just making boiled eggs. I'll pack some of those. I know they're your favorite."

Ronald sidled up to me. "You have time for a game of checkers, I think."

"Do I?" I asked Sieglinde.

She slammed her book shut and jumped to her feet. "Nope. I'm ready."

We pulled on our jackets and set off for the Zwarte Pad, which wound its way through the dunes, past the Kurhaus, and to the shop-lined boulevard. After a lovely walk past the Pier, we eventually sat on the beach to enjoy our food.

"Mmm, that was delicious. The smell of salt in the air makes everything taste so good." Meta leaned back on her elbows.

Sieglinde wiped her mouth and got to her feet. "I saw some nice seashells back there. I'm just going to pick some up. Be back soon."

My grateful eyes followed her before I turned to Meta, who was smirking. Seashells weren't exactly unusual on the beach. It appeared they'd made an arrangement so Meta and I could have some time alone.

Meta flopped onto her stomach next to me, her chin propped in her hands.

"Don't tell Siegie, but I think I really messed up this time, Frits. I may not even be allowed to graduate high school."

I'd been lying on my back with my hands behind my head but now rolled over onto my side to squint at her. "What did you do? You're nearly done!"

"*Ja*, I know, but I wanted to wear these to school." She sat up and wiggled her toes in her white sandals. "It's been so hot."

"*Ja*, and…?"

"Well, it's a Catholic school, so that wasn't allowed, at least not without socks. As if Jesus wore socks!"

"So, what happened?"

"I was also late that day, and everyone saw me because there was an assembly, and the principal kicked me out of school." Meta stopped for a breath before continuing. "I might have told him what Jesus wore."

I tried to hold back my chuckles, but they escaped.

"It's not funny, Frits! Mamma was so upset she was crying but didn't tell Pappa. Thank goodness!"

I wiped the tears from my cheeks before asking, "What are you going to do?"

"Luckily, my teacher likes me. He said I can study at his house for the remaining weeks. His daughter will bring me the work. But I'm still not sure I'll pass the government exams."

I shook my head. "Metì, that was a foolish stunt, but you're the smartest girl I know. You'll pass. Don't worry."

Meta sighed. "I hope so. Anyway, can you come to church with us tomorrow? Are you free?"

I shook my head. "I don't like the Catholic church. They're forever laying down the law, and nobody gets to give me orders!"

"Our priest is nice—well, he did tell Mamma and Pappa that they should have another baby right after the war ended, but except for that... You know, he's a widower and has two kids of his own. Please come! The music is lovely!"

"*Nee.*" I crossed my arms over my chest. "I don't believe in the Catholic God, and I don't want to pretend."

Meta jumped to her feet. "Oh, there's Siegie coming. It's probably getting late, and I want to pick some flowers on our way home."

Over the next few weeks, I saw very little of Meta. She was preparing for her exams. Finally, I couldn't stay away any longer and stopped by her house.

"Frits, I'm so nervous," she whispered as we stood on the balcony, allegedly to admire the garden she planted on the shed's roof. "I feel sick! What if my mind goes blank? What if..."

"Metì, lieveling (darling), stop worrying. You've been studying every day, so you'll be fine. And, if you get anxious during the test, remember: I'll be waiting for you just outside the building."

Meta's bright blue eyes grew round. "You will? But it's a workday."

"I'll take a day off. Where else would I be?"

"What are you two doing out there?" Pappa's deep voice made Meta jump. "Come in and join us."

"Yes, Pappa."

The dreaded day arrived. I met Meta at the Malieveld, and we walked hand-in-hand until it was time for her to go in for the written exams. I squeezed her ice-cold fingers and whispered, "I believe in you."

She nodded wordlessly, straightened her shoulders, and walked through the doors into the red brick building.

While Meta was inside, I stood by my bicycle, eyes fastened on where she'd entered. I may even have said a prayer or two. Just in case.

At lunchtime, the doors opened, and the frazzled candidates emerged like an ocean wave. Meta's anxious eyes sought me out.

"Meti! Here!" I waved as I forced my way upstream. "How was it?"

"It was easy! I think I did well." Meta did a little twirl.

"Great! Come on. Let's find a place to sit. I brought some bread and cheese for lunch."

Her face fell. "I really can't eat. What if I mess up the oral exam?"

"You need to…" No, that wouldn't work. It was obvious Meta was much too tense for food. "Let's go for a walk in *het bos*. We have an hour; let's use it!"

I took her hand, and leaving the crowd behind, we strolled through the nearby trees, listening to the birdsong and enjoying the gentle rustle of leaves. Coming across a bench that was almost invisible from the path, I led Meta to sit, and we rested in contented silence.

I felt I should say something, but nothing came to mind, so I acted on my instincts. I pulled my girlfriend into my arms, and with my heart beating so loudly I was sure she could hear it, I touched her lips with my own. To my astonishment, she didn't resist but put her head on my shoulder and nestled closer.

When Meta, with a grin on her face, returned for her oral exam, I stood waiting again. I knew she was being questioned in a group with five other candidates, but wasn't worried. One of Meta's strongest suits was the "gift of gab." She could talk her way through anything. I grinned just thinking about it.

At long last, the doors opened again. Meta emerged out of the middle of a group of excited classmates. Her family was also waiting by then, and we all joined her. The results would be posted in an hour.

"How do you think I did?" Meta's hands twisted together.

Mamma stroked her hair. "I'm sure you did fine. Calm down, schatje."

Although I couldn't touch her with her parents present, Meta's eyes sought mine out. I winked, even while experiencing a pang. I wished my mother was just a little bit like Meta's.

Finally, a man in a black cape posted the results to the board, and we crowded around to see.

Sieglinde was the first to spot her name. "Meta, you passed the A exams! With flying colors!"

"Let me see! I did!" Meta's eyes were shining. "So much for the principal!"

I cleared my throat to warn her that the self-same man was approaching.

"Congratulations, Meta," he intoned. "You understand I had to do what I did, but I'm glad you passed, anyway."

Pappa frowned. "Pretty sure I don't want to know what that was all about."

"Nothing important," Mamma responded with a smile.

Meta was a high school graduate.

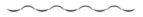

Gradually, as I gained their trust, Pappa and Mamma permitted Meta and me to spend time alone—outside and in public, of course. We'd walk in Westbroekpark, the Scheveningse bosjes, and the Frankenslag where I worked. Since walking provided the double benefit of not having to look into her eyes and nobody being able to hear, I opened up all about my sorry life, hoping against hope that Meta would still like me. After all, I figured, some of it was my own fault.

I spilled the story of being born in the Congo before moving to the Netherlands because Papa got sick and how I missed the boys. I shared about being put into a children's home, where I had to polish shoes every week, keep the *kachel* full of coal, and gather wood. I didn't tell her the full extent of how I was beaten because I remembered my decision to forgive. Meta never pulled her hand out of mine. Surely, that was a hopeful sign.

When my words slowed, Meta pulled me to a standstill. There was fire in her eyes. "The sisters are terrible people! Despicable!"

I shook my head. "*Nee,* I don't think they were so bad, at least not Zuster Deenik. They were harsh, but with the benefit of hindsight, I respect them. After all, I wasn't exactly an amiable child—at least, that's what Moeder tells me. She says I'm difficult."

"Hmmph! Don't get me started on her. I can't even imagine giving my children away!" Caught up in the dream, Meta gave a little twirl, her eyes now sparkling. "Children. I want at least a dozen."

"As long as I don't have to polish their shoes…"

Meta put her hands on her hips. "Well, if we get married and have children, they will wear shoes, and they will need polishing. So, whatever do you mean?"

I groaned. Meta sometimes had trouble understanding my sense of humor. "Never mind. So, did I tell you I got a raise at work? Now I can start paying Moeder back faster. Of course, there's nothing left for clothing or even toothpaste, but I guess soap will work."

"Yuck! We used salt during the war. I think that'd be better than soap."

I filed that piece of information away for the future. It was good that I did.

Meta (17) as she was when Frits met her, 1952. (top)

Frits on his bicycle, 1952. (bottom)

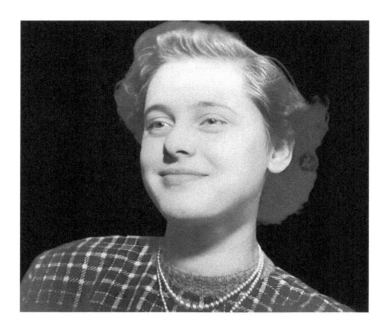

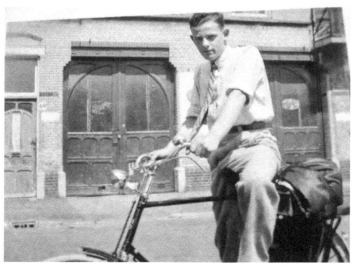

12

THE MILITARY

1953 Early in February, I received a letter in a very official-looking envelope. I opened it with trembling fingers. Since I was no longer in college, I was eligible for conscription into military service but had been hoping they wouldn't remember me. They did. The letter stated that starting on April 9, I would have to serve my country's army. I had no choice; it was mandatory. I would have to obey their orders on their timetable. Two months of freedom left; the clock was ticking.

I pulled the ham radio transmitter I'd built from under my bed and listened for my old friend. He was on! "Hey Henk, Frits here. How's your life today?"

By pressing the button on the receiver, I could hear his response amid the static. "I'm not working today, so that's good. But soon, it'll stink. I just received a letter from the army. I have to do my time."

I groaned. "Me, too. That's why I called. I guess we're going to be soldiers."

"Yeah, unfortunately. My problem is that I don't know what my family will do without me."

"I'm sorry, buddy. On the bright side, if there is one, at least we're no longer at war. Even better, I heard they'll pay us 49 cents daily—I'll be rich! Not you, of course, since you'll have to send it to your family."

"Enough for an entire pack of cigarettes or some chewing gum. Not both, of course. Can't be greedy."

I laughed. "Maybe we'll be in the same troop. Either way, we can stay in touch like this."

"Let's go celebrate our 'luck.' Meet me in the dunes? I could use some fresh air, exercise, and distraction."

"Yup, I'm free. For now, at least. See you there."

I grabbed my bicycle, and the sea breeze was soon ruffling my hair. After a brisk ride, I bade Henk farewell and rode to Meta's house. I had to break the news to her.

I hadn't even touched the doorbell when Meta opened the door, dressed in a red plaid skirt and a white woolen sweater. "I was sitting by the window and saw you riding up," she explained. "Why are you here?"

"I have something important to tell you."

"Everyone is in the living room, so let's sit here." Meta sat on the freshly scrubbed front stoop with her hands clasped in front of her knees.

Joining her, I pulled the letter out of my pocket and passed it over. "I've been conscripted."

Meta's eyes scanned the paper. "April 9," she murmured. "In Ede!" She sighed. "You'll be very far away, Freddy. I'm going to miss you so much!"

"And I'll miss you. But we can write and visit." I carefully put my arm around her, always mindful of the neighbors' and the *zedenpolitie's* (morality police's) watchful eyes.

Meta shook her head. "I won't be able to visit. The train is too expensive, and my bike broke. I even have to walk to work."

I drew my eyebrows together. "Why didn't you tell me? Let me look at it. Maybe I can fix it."

After an hour of tinkering, I realized the bicycle was beyond repair. The following week, all my savings in hand, I visited the bicycle shop. Then, with Sieglinde's help, I exchanged Meta's broken bike for a brand-new one. After all, a man has to take care of his girl.

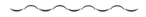

With Papa's *koffer* in hand, I hugged Meta goodbye and boarded the train to report to the Elias Beekman Kazerne (base). A flock of sheep caught my eye on the way, and I contemplated the fact that the goal of basic training was to turn us into sheep: fully prepared, mindlessly obedient, killing machine sheep. I knew that a trained army with soldiers who don't think for themselves is vital when at war, but was woefully aware that if the drill sergeant issued nonsensical orders, I would struggle. Would I be able to fake total compliance for 16 months? And if I couldn't, what then?

As soon as I had settled in the barracks, I wrote to Meta.

Dear Meta,

I just bought this stationery in the canteen. It was bursting with soldiers.

I am already class senior at the moment, and at the same time appointed by another non-commissioned officer as chamber guard. So, they seem to see something in me.

I haven't been to the doctor yet, maybe tomorrow. I did have to fill out some kind of medical form that asked if my feet were bothering me, so I answered *ja*.

Would you please send me the key to the padlock? You know which one is mine.

I am exhausted and am now going to lie down on my cot. I am writing only to you. Vader and Moeder, and the Family Verbeek will come tomorrow.

Keep courage, Metì, and a kiss from Frits.

The punishing schedule, getting up at 5:30 am, an hour of physical training, and then breakfast, began the very next morning. I was used to a regimented life at *het kindertehuis*, so the routine didn't trouble me as much as it did some men. Besides, swimming in the ocean had already rendered me very fit. After a physical, where the physician complained about my flat feet (as if I could do something about them), I was issued a military ID and given my rifle, a cotton summer uniform, a dress uniform for Sundays, a woolen winter uniform, and army boots, albeit a size too large. It was more clothing than I'd had since I lived in the Congo!

I was assigned to the 2nd regiment, 4th company, 2nd battalion, 3rd platoon, and 2nd class. There were only 20 men in that class, and because I'd had some post-secondary education and was a little older than the others, the colonel put me in charge. I hoped he wouldn't come to regret that decision.

On Sunday morning, the drill sergeant, Sergeant Roep, informed us that all soldiers have to go to church, whether to a Roman Catholic or a Protestant one. I heaved a sigh. Why was religion forced down my throat everywhere I went? A major marched those of us who preferred the latter to the Protestant church, where he gave a talk that was certainly not a sermon. In fact, there was no mention of religion.

I leaned toward the soldier next to me. "Who is he, and where's the minister?"

"He's the chaplain."

My eyebrows ascended into my forehead. "It sounds like he doesn't believe in God."

"Who knows? All I know is he's boring!"

Once we were back on base, they relegated my class to a room where we were to remain for the rest of the day. The sheep were in their pen.

"Hey, Evenblij!"

I stopped filling in my crossword puzzle and turned to Hans Wildemast, the soldier with whom I shared a bedroom. "Yes?"

"What do you think about us being a unique class, one that has some standards?"

The noise level in the room dropped as the others listened in to what I would decide. I was, after all, the sheepdog, if you like.

I pursed my lips and nodded slowly. "Like what?"

"Well, let's agree not to drink too much."

The other soldiers laughed until I put up my hand. "That sounds extremely sensible, Wildemast, but let's do more."

One man seated near me looked slightly alarmed. "Seriously?"

I nodded. I knew what Meta would wish for my behavior. "We'll agree to stay upright and self-disciplined. No cursing, womanizing, or drinking too much. We'll sleep as soon as we go to bed, and we'll help each other."

Some soldiers grumbled, but agreement came quickly.

The next day, we had an inspection, which I had to oversee.

"Men, go sit on the bench," I bellowed. They obeyed. The idea of making them do something ridiculous flashed through my mind, but I resisted the temptation. I even schooled my features to show no sign of my thoughts.

Once the lieutenant came in, I commanded, "In order." They all stood up.

"Class!" They all pulled their clothing straight.

"Attention!" Everyone stood to attention.

Next, I turned myself around and marched to the lieutenant. Once I was two steps away from him, I saluted.

After walking up and down the line, the officer commanded, "Bring the class at ease and let them sit."

I turned and barked at the class, and the sheep obeyed. Of course, they had no choice, and given my dislike of being ordered around, I was delighted it was me giving the orders!

During the next couple of weeks, the physical training program intensified. It started with running across the base without a top, regardless of the weather. It progressed to lifting weights, doing pushups, marching, and even scaling an obstacle course.

I pressed my lips together as my blistered feet screamed their protests after walking 25 km in old socks and new, too-big boots. Although I was used to physical pain, I remembered that the doctor had noted my flat feet and decided to alert him to the problem I was having. He examined my feet, listened to my chest, and then said, "Get dressed and walk on." No help there.

Sergeant Roep stood with his arms across his pigeon chest. "Girls, give me 25 more push-ups." We'd already completed 200.

An emaciated man attempted to obey, his arms trembling with the effort, but he was forced to give up after two.

"Well, look at the weakling! Maybe he expects me to help?" Sergeant Roep kicked the soldier's side.

My eyes narrowed. I hated bullies! My childhood had rendered me pretty immune to verbal abuse, and because I didn't respect him, his words just washed over me. It was difficult to say nothing about this kind of behavior, but I knew it would only stoke his fire.

Once the little man deemed us ready, we moved on to the next part of the training: use of our rifles, navigation, and breaking codes. Since puzzles of all kinds fascinated me, I quickly became engrossed in the latter two.

Then came the final part of the training.

"Men, today you're going to learn to crawl," Sergeant Roep intoned.

Wildemast and I exchanged glances. What could he mean? Even babies know how to crawl!

Sergeant Roep smirked before leading us through streaming rain and howling wind to a field. "Get down on your bellies and move from here to the other end of the field. Make sure you keep your heads and backsides down."

My class lay down on the muddy ground as instructed, preparing to go once we received the order.

Suddenly, we heard gunfire. Sweat rolled into my eyes as the sound threw me back into the incident in Driebergen. The all-too-familiar feeling of panic ensued, but I knew now was not the time. Blinking to clear my vision, I turned my head to the side and saw two lines of soldiers shooting live ammunition across the field where we were meant to crawl. Their guns were only 40 cm (16 in) above ground level. My terrified eyes clashed with Wildemast's, who winked, of all things.

"Heads down. And go!" Sergeant Roep screamed, his spit flying in all directions. I was glad I was nowhere near the human saliva machine.

"*Stommerik* (dumbass)," I heard Wildemast mutter.

I briefly considered rebelling against this senseless and dangerous exercise, but not for long. If they were willing to wound, possibly fatally, those who were trying and failing to stay down, they would certainly kill anyone who refused to try. Keeping myself as low to the soggy ground as possible, I obeyed, making a mental note to speak with Wildemast about his language.

Each week built on the last until we sheep were supposedly a team fit for fighting. By nightfall, we fell into our cold, rock-hard bunks with their equally thin pillows and slept like the dead.

Actually, apart from one issue, I didn't do too badly at basic training. The offending drill comprised being unexpectedly roused out of a deep sleep in the middle of the night. Whenever I was awoken, I jumped up and punched whoever was nearby. This was definitely frowned upon, but no matter how much I was disciplined, it didn't change. And it was always my fault. A gift from my childhood.

My army experience, indeed my life, often reminded me of the poem by Guido Gezelle. While in the army, I adopted it as my motto.

Het leven is een strijdbanier,	Life is a battle banner,
Door goede en kwade dagen,	Through good and bad days,
Gescheurd, gevlekt, ontvallen schier,	Torn, soiled, almost destroyed,
	Carried valiantly forward.
Kloekmoedig voorwaards gedragen	

~~~~~~

"Evenblij, come to my office at 14:00 hours."

I saluted Colonel Bazig while narrowing my eyes. What could this order be about? Although I was frequently disciplined for lack of compliance, there hadn't been any recent incidents. "Yes, sir."

I knocked on the colonel's door once my work for the day was complete and entered when he responded. He was seated at a long desk, but I remained standing with my hands clasped tightly behind my back.

"Evenblij, we've been watching you, how you handle the accounts, your cartography skills, and more. I also see that you did very well on the tests you took during basic training, maybe because you have a year of college under your belt."

Here, he paused, evidently expecting a response. "Thank you, sir."

Colonel Bazig nodded and continued, "Therefore, I have great news for you. We decided that you are officer material. Congratulations! You'll begin training tomorrow." He picked up his pencil, evidently thinking the conversation was over.

"Sir, with respect, that's my decision. I don't want to be an officer. Being in the army is not my life's goal."

The man's eyebrows drew together. "Consider carefully. As part of this, you'd be sent to college. This would be a way for you to complete your training at MTS and have a job coming out."

It was a tempting offer. I briefly closed my eyes. The memory of the soldiers who evaluated Jan and me before taking my cousins, Keetie and the other Jewish children to their deaths would always haunt me. Of course, those men were Germans, but basic training had drilled into me that all soldiers have to obey their commanding officers. I neither wanted to kill someone nor tell someone else to do it. Shaking my head, I repeated what I'd said. "I don't want to be in the army."

Colonel Bazig's nostrils flared. "You're making the wrong decision. Think it over tonight, and we'll talk again tomorrow."

The flush on his face told me now was not the time to argue. But no matter what they offered me, I knew I neither wanted someone else to own me nor to be forced to do what another man decided was right. I also didn't want to do that to others. The army was definitely not the place for me.

The next evening, I was again summoned to Colonel Bazig's room, now facing a row of uniformed, stern-faced men, all seated behind a long table. I almost expected to see a Rolodex in front of them. "Well, Evenblij? Have you come to your senses?"

"*Nee,* sir…I mean, yes, sir. *Ja,* I am in my right mind, and, *nee,* I don't want to t…t…train to be an officer. Sir." I saluted smartly.

Colonel Bazig rose to his feet, sucking the air out of the room before his inevitable explosion. "Idiot! You think you don't want to be here? Well, I have news for you. Your time as a conscript has just changed from 16 to 22 months." He snapped his fingers to emphasize the point. "And, unless you come to your senses, I'll personally make sure you never increase in rank beyond corporal. Now get out of our sight!"

I again saluted sharply and turned on my heel, rolling my eyes once my back was turned. I knew whom I considered an idiot, and it wasn't me.

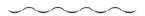

Wildemast and I were posted to Middelburg in Zeeland, 75 miles from Scheveningen, in June. Frequent letters would just not be enough for Meta and me, but the army forbade visits. Regardless, we arranged that she would take the train and stay for a couple of days. What they didn't know…

When Meta arrived on base, Wildemast was in the sentry box on guard duty. He wasn't allowed to speak, smile, or react, but he did one of his famous bird calls to tell her it was safe to approach and alert me to her presence.

I came out of the office, and there she was, pretty as a picture with her cornflower blue eyes and windblown cheeks. Nobody apart from my friend was around, so I gave her a quick hug.

"Hey, Meta, it sure was good of you to come see me," Wildemast joked.

Meta giggled but joined right in. "Well, you know, it's better than nothing, even if this guy had to be here." She poked me in the arm.

Just then, Sergeant Zweterig came striding around the corner, presumably to check up on the difficult soldier—me.

"Quick, Meta!" Wildemast shoved her behind him and swiftly stood at attention. Sergeant Zweterig strode past him without a glance, following me as I disappeared into the office.

When he finally finished our conversation and left, Meta tapped my rather substantial friend on his back.

"Coast is clear," Wildemast whispered without moving his lips. "Go on into the office. I'll keep watch."

That was just as well because my unusual cooperativity had made my archnemesis suspicious. Sergeant Zweterig doubled back just after Meta joined me. Another friend, who was watching Wildemast for signals, knocked on the wall to alert Meta and me to the danger. In no time, I secreted her into the cupboard behind the *kachel*, the one where we stored ammunition.

Sergeant Zweterig flung the door open, and his beady eyes peered into every corner, his odor filling the room. I stood at attention, carefully schooling my face to not show my thoughts. Finally, after asking several pointless questions, he gave up. Meta, who by then had been in the gun closet, crouched among live ammunition for quite a time, crept out. She looked decidedly less vivacious than when she'd entered.

That night, Meta took Wildemast's bunk in my room, and we were able to talk until the early hours. He slept on the floor of the office. It was still dark when we heard a knock on the door. Meta gasped and dove under her bed, sure that we'd been caught, even if we'd only been sleeping. I pretended to stretch and yawn loudly as if I'd just woken up. I figured Wildemast would be the one to get in trouble. After all, he wasn't in bed where he should have been!

The door swung open, and the delicious smell of coffee filled the room. It was only Wildemast, bearing our breakfast in his hands.

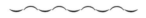

Strolling hand-in-hand with Meta through the forest near Driebergen, my heart swelled with happiness. Yes, I was in the army but it was temporary. And today, sunlight dappled the forest floor; the leaves were beginning to turn color, and the breeze was fragrant. I stopped to gaze at the bundle of energy next to me and realized that I was head-over-heels in love for the first time in my life.

Immediately, panic took hold, and my mind flashed to the many people I'd loved and lost: the boys, Papa, Keetie, and my cousins. Even Jan was kind of gone, being almost totally withdrawn into himself. Would Meta leave, too? My chest started aching, and I felt a prick behind my eyes. Nonetheless, that night I carefully typed out a note to my beloved.

The next time I saw Meta, I had the letter in my pocket. I fingered it anxiously. Did I dare give it to her? I had to take a chance. I just had to. I had to give her the rather discolored piece of paper, which I'd folded many times in my anxiety. I held it out, my hand visibly trembling. "This is for you, Metì."

"Oh, thanks?" Meta curiously took the paper and read it several times.

> My Dearest Meta Antonia Bisschop,
> It will be my pleasure to offer you my hand in this way. I will not even ask for yours anymore, for you will not give it, anyway.
>
> > Your dearly loving,
> > D.pl.Sold. F. Evenbly
> > Leggno. 33.05.03.094,
> > 2-1 C.O.A.K.
> > Kazerne Koningstraat,
> > MIDDELBURG

She tilted her head and scrunched up her nose. "This is a joke. Right?"

"Well, kind of. Not really." I stuffed my hands into my pockets to stop them from twirling.

Meta frowned briefly before her laughing eyes met mine. "Whatever do you mean by it, Freddy? You're so weird sometimes. Oh, look at that sweet little chipmunk." She stuffed the paper in her pocket before running to look closer, picking a few wildflowers on the way.

I grinned. It was sometimes challenging to keep her on topic. "Lieveling, wait! I have a question: will you *be* with me?"

Meta sighed and pushed away the strands of nut-brown hair that the wind had blown into her eyes. "I'm with you already. I'm right here."

I took a deep breath and continued. After all, I'd gone this far. "I know that if I ask you to marry me, you probably won't agree. So, I'm asking, will you be with me? And never, ever leave me?"

Her eyes widened as she squeaked, "You want to marry me?"

"Well, not yet. I'm still in the army, but *ja*...one day."

I nearly fell over as Meta threw herself into my arms, scattering flowers all around us. "*Ja, ja, ja, ja*! I love you, Freddy!"

Now, as I held her tight, the tears could no longer be contained. It was September 6, and I was engaged to the most amazing girl in the world. She would never leave me. How could that even be true? Elation filled all the empty places in my soul.

"Come on, Metì, let's carve our initials into the Swiss Bridge. Then everyone will know we're in love!"

"Not my parents. You'll have to ask Pappa for my hand." Meta got down on one knee to mime what she thought I should do.

I chuckled. "And you, Mademoiselle, will have to ask Moeder for mine."

Meta gasped, "Don't even joke about that! She's terrifying."

"*Ja*, she is. But, for now, where should we put our initials?"

"Mmm, right here. Next to this tree. FE+MAB"

When I next had leave, I took the train to the Verbeeks, picked up my bike, and rode it to the Leeuwardensestraat. I was just about to press the doorbell when I realized the shouting I could hear was coming from Meta's home.

"Children cost money! What in the world do you expect me to do?"

D*amn it! Just spend less! I can't possibly pick up more work. And we have to pay down the debt from Corrie's illness."

"I'm doing my best. I'm even working at the hairdresser. But maybe I should just throw myself into the ocean! It'd be better than living here with you."

I gulped and rang, anyway. The voices ceased immediately, and Meta met me at the bottom of the stairs.

"Umm, is everything okay?"

"Yeah, they argue a lot. My sister Corrie's treatments were expensive; now they're worried about money. They do love each other, but both my parents have tempers. I hate it!"

I was silent for a few minutes, mulling this over. I never wanted Meta to experience anything she "hates" again, so I determined to ensure money was never a stressor in our marriage. "Is this a good time to talk to them about us?"

Meta shrugged. "Let's give Mamma a few minutes to get over her hysterics. Then, it'll be fine."

"Okay, we'll walk around the block before going in."

When we returned to the house, Meta rang the bell as if she were a visitor, just in case. Siegie came down, looking like the cat who got the cream. Evidently, Meta had shared her news with her sister. "Good luck," she whispered, making me worry I might need it.

I didn't. The only sign of their argument was Mamma's reddened eyes. Once Meta's parents had been assured that we wouldn't marry until I had a job where I could support her, they enthusiastically welcomed me to the family. Mamma even said I would be her son once we married, just as much as Meta was her daughter. Imagine that! I would have a mother who acted like one.

Moeder was my next stop, and her response was very different. I was glad that I didn't bring Meta. "Frits, you're not thinking with your head. It's probably because you're much too young to make this kind of decision."

I opened my mouth, and Moeder held up a hand to stop me from speaking.

"Consider! Meta's family is working-class." She wrinkled her nose as if detecting a foul odor. "You need a girl with money, one who's worthy of our family."

I snorted. "Her family is worth a million of ours, Moeder. You know, they actually love each other!"

Moeder ignored my outburst. "If you marry her, you'll be sorry. Mark my words."

After slamming the door on my way out, I cycled to Meta's house, where plans were underfoot.

"I hope we can have the engagement party at Frits's mother's and stepfather's home—it's big enough to hold a lot of people. Mevrouw Ouwerkerk tried to dissuade me from marrying Frits, but it didn't work. Since she knows that, I expect she'll come around."

I cleared my throat. "Moeder does love showing off her elegant home."

Meta rolled her eyes before continuing. "We'll invite all our friends and relatives, and my dress will be as blue as the sky."

Sieglinde laughed. "Of course. To match your eyes. You'll be a beautiful lady."

"Oh, *ja,*" Meta simpered in a sophisticated lady's voice, pretending to adjust her hair.

I smiled before pulling a round pink vase filled with fragrant stephanotis from behind my back. "My lady," I said, executing a courtly bow. "Now, let's go buy our rings and have them inscribed with our names and the date we got engaged."

Meta sighed. "Freddy, I'm crazy about you. I never thought this kind of beautiful love was possible, and now we're actually living it."

Although I couldn't express myself like she did, my heart agreed. The day that I put that simple gold band on the third finger of Meta's right hand, and she put one on mine, was the proudest day of my life so far.

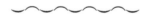

Sinterklaas was approaching, and while I wasn't interested in receiving gifts, I was excited because the army said we would be allowed to visit family on December 6. I would not be going to see Moeder.

I stared at the coins I'd saved. What could I give Meta? And, even if I could afford something, would she like it? I knew I wasn't good at choosing gifts and kind of wished I could ask her to do it for me. Maybe I would, once we were married.

The main street shops were full of Sinterklaas wares but provided me with little inspiration. Clasping my hands behind my back, I carried on walking until I came to a place that sold clothing. A smile teased the corners of my mouth. How often did Meta talk about what so-and-so was wearing, what she and Siegie were knitting for Ronald, and the sky-blue dress she dreamed of making for herself?

"Come in, meneer. Is there something that caught your eye?"

Fingering the pretty blue scarf on the display nearest the door, I responded. "*Ja*, I think my fiancé would like this. Would you, I mean, if you were a girl?"

The sales lady laughed. "I am a girl, but I know what you meant. What color are your fiancé's eyes?"

"Oh, they're the prettiest blue you can imagine."

"Then this scarf is the very thing. It'll bring out the blue in her eyes."

I gave a decisive nod. "Wrap it up, *alstublieft*."

Back at the barracks, I carefully wrapped my gift in a long tube. Then, with my tongue sticking out of the side of my mouth as it was wont to do, I wrote a poem. Once done, I carefully cut out each line and pasted them around the tube, making a spiral. *Ja,* that looked amazing.

But would it be enough? Buying more wasn't an option—I'd used all my savings on the scarf and a small chocolate "M." With my head pillowed on my hand and my elbow on the table, I thought hard enough to give myself a headache.

Suddenly, I straightened up, almost as if Zuster Dermout had entered the room. What a great idea! I'd been making radios since I was 12. Perhaps Meta would like me to build one for her. Once I'd saved a few more guilders, we could shop for the radio tubes together. This was a pursuit I always enjoyed, so surely, she would love it, too. I could build the radio in a cigar box and paint it red. After carefully drawing a radio and adding the paper to my gift, I was done.

At 5:00 on Sinterklaas, dressed in my army uniform, I rang the doorbell at Leeuwardensestraat 1. The door swung open when Meta pulled the rope at the top, and I mounted the steep stairs to her home in three leaps. Of course, kissing my fiancé technically wasn't allowed, but I pulled her into my arms for a warm hug before bestowing a quick peck on her lips. No one was looking.

After dinner, the gifts came out. Ronald and Siegie drew near to watch as Meta undid the tube and read out my poem. It talked about how Sinterklaas said dark chocolate letters with hazelnuts were scarce. I wrote that I'd begged him, so he and Piet searched everywhere and finally found a small one. The poem ended with advising her to eat the letter quickly. It wasn't exactly a van Alphen, but the way she carefully folded the wrapping paper and set it in a safe place told me she was delighted. It seemed she liked the poem better than the scarf and the chocolate. Would I ever understand women?

"There's also this," I said, thrusting the folded drawing in her direction.

Meta's cheeks turned a pretty pink. "First, open the gift I made for you." She handed me a parcel wrapped in notebook paper, which she had colored so it appeared to be covered with flowers.

After pretending to smell the flowers and declaring them oh-so-fragrant, I carefully unpicked the tape to reveal--a blue and gray hand-knitted scarf. I immediately put it around my neck before striking a pose.

Siegie giggled. "Very nice! And you'll match!"

Unable to wait, I thrust my next gift into Meta's hand. "Open this now!" I leaned forward, wanting to see her face, when she realized what a fantastic present I planned to make her.

"Oh wow!" Meta's tone belied her words. "You're going to build me a red radio? But how will it work? Will it be complicated? Will I be able to use it?" Meta frowned as she stared at the drawing.

My heart sank. Of course. My new fiancé was quite technologically disabled. She must be. I couldn't imagine that she wouldn't share my interest in it! Never mind. The radio wouldn't be challenging to use, and it'd be fun to teach her. Or so I thought.

"Come sit. It's time for dinner." Mamma graciously waved her hand toward the beautifully set table in the middle of the living room.

Pappa stubbed out his cigarette and took the chair at the head of the table. Mamma was seated on the opposite end, nearest to the kitchen. "Come sit here next to me, Frits." Pappa indicated the place on his right, but I sat on his left. I always wanted Meta on my left, nearest to my heart. He looked a bit confused, but Meta just grinned. She knew. I looked around the small, clean, cozy room with its smiling faces. What was Moeder complaining about?

It was late when Meta accompanied me to the door. "When will I see you again?" She was twisting her skirt between her fingers.

"They told us we have Christmas Day off, so I hope I can come then."

"How early can you get here? Mamma and Sieglinde are singing in the choir at church. The music is always so beautiful! Will you be in time for the service?"

I chuckled. "Not if I can help it. I can barely stand the Protestant services in the army; I certainly won't be able to tolerate a Catholic one."

Meta's eyes welled up with tears. "*Alsjeblieft*?"

"You know I hate being forced. *Nee*!"

Meta sighed. "Well, it'll just be good to see you." She stood on her toes to peck my cheek.

As I walked away, my stomach hurt. I was glad she always backed down instead of fighting me but refusing her request made me feel so evil.

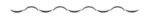

The army completed their assessment of my capabilities and decided I was good at math. It didn't take a genius to figure that out! I was assigned to the Zware Transport Compagnie, where I counted out the soldiers' meager wages, placed the money in paper bags, and drove a jeep to deliver the salaries. A couple of other soldiers always accompanied me, just in case I should decide to abscond with the riches! It was a job I relished, given that I could both dabble in accounting and indulge in the occasional illicit escapade.

Today my route would go through Den Haag, where Meta now worked in the office of a paint factory, N.V. Verf-En VernisFabriek on the Binckhorstlaan. Technically, of course, we weren't allowed to make private stops, but since I was the eldest and the driver, I planned on doing just that. Wildemast and the other soldiers would never say a word.

We arrived at the factory to find the gated parking lot manned by an aged gatekeeper. Fortunately, I knew his wife liked Meta so much that she frequently invited her into the gatehouse. That should help.

"Do you have business at the factory?" the old man croaked.

"Yes, I'm here to see my fiancé, Meta Bisschop."

"Ah, a lovely young woman that. Come in." The gate slowly opened for us, and we entered a nearly empty parking lot. Most people cycled to work.

It was a little early for the lunch break, and the gatekeeper again had his head in the newspaper, so I spent some time playing. My buddies shouted with laughter as I made donuts in the army jeep, aided by the icy conditions.

Finally, Meta appeared, bundled in her coat and laden with five warm bottles of milk.

"How did you get these, schatje?" I asked.

"The factory provides the workers with milk because it protects them from the leaded paint fumes. Everyone always puts their bottles on the huge *kachel* to heat up in time for their lunch. But the factory workers enjoyed your amazing show so much that a few of them came to our building. They told us they were donating their milk as payment."

"Sure wish they could have seen me driving on the dike! We were virtually sideways," I chuckled.

"And I nearly lost my breakfast." Wildemast pointed his finger toward his open mouth and made a gagging noise.

Meta shook her head before taking a seat next to me. "This is why the recruits love you and the officers hate you."

I pulled up our kit from the back to share among the men and Meta, and we enjoyed Edam cheese sandwiches with warm milk. Time flew until the city clock chimed the hour.

Meta gave a start. "Oh, I need to go; my break is over." With a flurry of skirts, my fiancé disappeared, and with a wave to the gatekeeper, we drove on.

When we arrived at the next base, a group of soldiers was waiting for us, their eyes sparkling.

"Frits, we know your job is vital, so we provided you with a suitable desk and chair. Come with us."

My eyebrows drew together. Passing out a few paper bags didn't strictly require the use of an office.

The tallest soldier opened the door to the storage room with a flourish before bowing in an exaggerated manner. "Welcome to your office, Sir Moneybags."

Mystified, I entered to find a desk and chair made entirely from hand grenades. "Oh, *bedankt*, kind sirs!" I gingerly placed my bags of money on the desk, sat on the explosive devices, and proceeded to pay everyone, much to the amusement of the recipients.

~~~~~~

1954 As the weather continued frigid, the sound of coughing in the barracks became commonplace. Like the nurses at het kindertehuis, the army officials believed exercising outdoors without a shirt was somehow beneficial to health. Given the apparent results, it was hardly a logical premise, but I knew arguing was pointless.

On a rainy day early in January, I awoke soaked with sweat, almost too weak to get out of bed. After stumbling through the morning exercises, the thought of breakfast was nauseating. "Sir," I said as I approached the sergeant, "I think I'm sick."

"Man up, Evenblij. Give me fifty pushups."

I fell to the ground and began, trembling and dripping with perspiration despite the icy wind. Screwing my eyes closed and pressing my lips together, I finished, having no desire to be punished for being obstinate. Again.

Finally, Saturday arrived. Although the weakness was almost overwhelming, I was determined not to miss out on the best part of my life: time with Meta. I left the base early, took the train to De Haag, stumbled to the Verbeeks from the station, and picked up my bike. Shaking with the effort of pedaling, I rode to the dunes where we'd agreed to meet. There, I had no choice but to sink down beside the path to catch my breath and wait for the pain in my lungs to subside. It was good to be a bit early, but I wondered what could be wrong with me. This felt like more than a cold!

There she was, her hair streaming behind her as she rode and her cheeks reddened by the wind. I struggled to my feet.

Alarm flared in Meta's eyes. "What's wrong, Freddy? You look terrible!" In no time, she had her hand on my forehead. "Oh my, you're burning up."

"I am? I don't feel very well, but expect I can manage, anyway."

Meta frowned. "I don't think so. Bicycling when you're this sick is a bad, bad idea. Come on. You can rest while I make you some tea sweetened with honey."

Too enervated to argue, I followed her home and collapsed onto the divan in their back room. Meta tucked a blanket around me, and I lay there motionless, only raising myself on one elbow when Meta brought my tea. I dozed until it was time to go. Meta helped me into my coat and then pressed some money into my hand. "Leave your bike here. You can't ride back."

Coughing too much to argue, I stuffed the coins into my pocket. She'd hung my bike on the hallway wall while I was sleeping, so with her help, I took the tram to the train station. Meta was right. There was no way I could have ridden even a short distance, let alone a long one.

Despite giving up the cigarette habit I'd picked up during my early days in the army, I remained ill for the rest of the winter. Night sweats, weakness, fevers, weight loss, and coughing became the story of my life. Of course, with the weather in the Netherlands, coughing all winter was pretty common. Nonetheless, on bad days, even the sergeant could see how ill I was. He actually allowed me to spend time in the sick bay! But they never tried to figure out what was wrong with me.

~~~~~~~~

Dear Frits,

It's all change in yours truly's life. You know I was working for the Foundation of Household and Family Education with a very nice boss—an older lady, of all things? She died. Another job, another dead boss. Not my doing, I assure you!

The job made me think. Why does our government spend money on nonsense, like knitting potholders? No answer to that one!

Now I'm going to sail around the world on a ship. Might as well, right? Sure hope nobody dies!

But first, I heard that you'll soon be 21. I think I'll stick around to see you become an adult. I'm wondering if it'll help.

Your boating brother, Jan

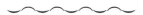

"Van den Broek, go to the barracks. You're drunk again."

The newly enlisted soldier I'd just called out pointed his wavering first finger in my direction. "Oh, hear what the big guy is saying."

"I've warned you repeatedly, and I won't say it again, Private."

Van den Broek rolled his eyes at me. "You're beginning to bore me, Evenblij."

His friends snickered, but at least he staggered toward his bunk.

I said nothing more to any of them but turned on my heel. I'd done some research on this insolent soldier. His father was a person with alcohol use disorder who'd been arrested in 1919, so he probably had a difficult childhood. But I knew from experience that was no excuse for inappropriate behavior. I would have to report him to prevent more insubordination from breaking out.

Van den Broek only got five days of detention, but it did the trick—both in bringing him into line and in earning me the reputation of a hard-ass.

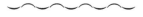

My 21st birthday was on a Monday, so Meta invited me to Moeder's house on Sunday. Since we became engaged, Moeder was always willing to host our gatherings. There was no more point in fighting that battle, and I suspected Vader doing the cooking and cleaning helped.

I jumped off my bike, slightly out of breath, not totally recovered from my extended spell of ill health. Meta, who'd been watching for me from Moeder's living room window, burst out of the front door and threw her arms around my neck. *"Hartelijk gefeliciteerd met je verjaardag!"*

Putting my hands on either side of her face, I drank in her rosy lips with my eyes before giving her a resounding kiss.

Meta gasped. "Frits! We're outside! What if someone is looking?"

"Let them look, and I hope they enjoy it. If I can't kiss my fiancé's lips on my birthday, when can I?" I did it again to prove the point.

Giggling, Meta grasped my hand and drew me up the stairs. "Just wait until you see."

Moeder and Vader's rowhouse had two big rooms on its main floor: the living room at the front and the dining room, where Moeder slept on a divan, at the back. Vader was relegated to the smaller bedroom on the third floor of the building. Both main rooms were lavishly decorated with flowers and happy birthday signs.

I turned around in astonishment. "Lieveling, this is beautiful. You're so good at making a place cozy—even a place like this!"

"Frits, you old dog! I thought I heard your voice." Jan sauntered into the living room with a grin.

"*Ja*, the handsome *broer* has arrived."

"Hmm, well, that's because the clever one was already here."

Vader cleared his throat. He really didn't understand brotherly joking. "Would anyone like *een borreltje* (alcoholic drink) before the guests arrive?"

Once we were seated, drink in hand, I raised my eyebrows at Meta, who understood my unspoken question. As was customary for her, her smile almost reached her ears. "I invited my sisters, Corrie's husband, Piet, and Siegie's boyfriend, Lou. Hans, Arie, Henk, and some other friends are also coming. But, before they arrive, I want to give you your gift. I can't wait!" She picked up a large rectangular package from the table and placed it in my hands.

I carefully opened the beautifully wrapped parcel to reveal a box from a local tailor. Meta had given me a brown woolen suit. I didn't have a suit or indeed any clothing apart from my uniforms. Buying even a new pair of pants on a soldier's salary was impossible.

I stroked the fabric and turned it over and over in my hands. This cost a fortune! Meta must have been saving for months, if not longer. Finally, I forced out some words. "Schatje, I don't know what to say."

Meta beamed. "Maybe you want to get changed before the other guests arrive. I put a clean shirt ready in Vader's bedroom."

As I got to my feet, Moeder's voice arrested me. "We also have a gift for you. Vader, pass this over, *alsjeblieft*."

Vader gave me a small box, which had obviously been professionally gift-wrapped. I opened it without enthusiasm to discover a very fitting, but not expensive, 21st birthday gift: a watch. "*Dank u wel*, Moeder and Vader."

Moeder pursed her lips. "It would've been more appropriate for Meta to get you the watch since a suit costs way too much."

Seeing Meta open her mouth, I shook my head at her. It wasn't worth arguing—it never was. "I'll wear them both and look quite the gentleman for the party."

"A gentleman maybe, but not as handsome as me!"

I rolled my eyes at Jan.

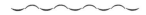

"Hey, Metì, next week my platoon will visit the fair in Ermelo. Do you want to come? Not Siegie. Just you. We'll have lots of chaperones. But you'd have to sleep near the base the night before."

Meta frowned. "I don't think I can. Pappa would never allow it!"

"You'd stay at a bed and breakfast in Ermelo."

Both of us were very aware of the *zedenpolitie*. They were always watching to be sure young people didn't spend time alone where no one could see them.

"That'd probably be okay," Meta said slowly. "I'll ask Pappa."

"Great! Come to my barracks an hour or two ahead of time, and my buddies and I will smuggle you onto the public bus so no officer will know you're with me. You know the soldiers all like you."

Meta's eyes lit up. She was always game to test the limits. "If Pappa agrees, I'll be there with bells on."

"Hmm, maybe leave the bells behind. They might attract unwanted attention."

The day went off without a hitch. Almost. Meta accompanied my platoon on the bus to and from the fair, and we had a great day. The problem was that it was also a hot, hot day.

In my opinion, one of the army's more ridiculous rules was that we were to look professional at all times. In other words, rolling up the sleeves of our uniforms was strictly forbidden. We did it anyway.

The bus was rocking with the sound of singing and laughing on the way back to base, and I tucked Meta into my side as we sat on the left in the middle of the bus. Suddenly, Meta leaped to her feet and emitted a most unladylike whistle, shocking me into silence.

"Quick, everyone! Roll down your sleeves. Someone is waiting in hiding over there—I saw him just now."

My friends hurriedly obliged, but I really wanted Meta to see I was every bit as courageous as she was. I left my sleeves rolled up.

As soon as I disembarked with my arm around Meta, one of the MPs shouted, "Corporal! Come over here. And is that a female person with you?"

Keeping Meta firmly by my side, I sauntered over to the man.

"Why did you bring the girl? I wanted to speak with you, not her. About your lack of professionalism." His face was almost puce with rage. Already.

"She's not just a girl. She's my fiancé!" I showed him my ring finger, offended by his implication that Meta was a woman of the street. "And, *ja,* I'll roll my sleeves down. Don't get all bent out of shape."

"Insolence! I'll be reporting you."

I wiped his saliva off my face before replying, "Then I'll see the report when you do. You see, I'm the administrator. All reports come across my desk."

"I'll make sure this one doesn't!" he sputtered.

Schooling my features to appear unconcerned, I questioned, "Why? I promise I'd make sure it'd go exactly where it belongs." As I spoke, I rolled my sleeves down and turned to walk away.

"Corporal, come back! I'm not used to being treated so disrespectfully. No salute, and you didn't even say '*Goedenavond,* sir!'"

By now, I was also becoming pretty irate, and it showed. I saluted the man in an exaggerated manner and drawled, "Is there any other order, Sergeant?"

"That isn't the way you address me!" By now, spittle was flying right and left.

I rolled my eyes at him and winked over my shoulder at Meta, who had backed away and stood with her mouth open.

The man snapped his fingers, and, in no time, I was slapped into handcuffs.

My sentence was solitary confinement, beginning on June 22 and lasting for ten days. Maybe it would have been less if I'd been drunk! I didn't mind all that much—except I missed the total solar eclipse on June 30, and they only reoccur in a given place approximately every 400 years. I figured that meant I probably wouldn't see another.

Frits (bottom left) in the army, 1953. (top)

Frits asks Meta to marry him through a typed note, 1953. (bottom)

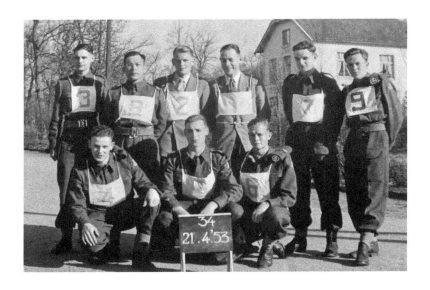

Hooggeachte Mejufrouw Meta Antonia Bisschop,

Het zal me hierbij een genoegen zijn U op deze wijze m'n hand aan
te bieden, om de Uwe vragen doe ik maar niet eens meer, want U geeft
hem toch niet.
      Uw innig lieflebbende

               D.pl.Sold. F.Evenblij,
               Leg.no. 33.05.03.094,
               2-I C.O.A.K.
               Kazerne Koningstraat,
               MIDDELBURG.

The report that led to Frits being given solitary confinement, 1954.

ORIGINEEL EXEMPLAAR

KONINKLIJKE MARECHAUSSEE
3e DIVISIE
DISTRICT   ZWOLLE
BRIGADE   HARDERWIJK

No.R.114 /54

R A P P O R T.

Op Zaterdag 19 Juni 1954 te omstreeks 22.40 uur, bevond ik,
FRANS VAN D IJ K,Wachtmeester le klasse der Koninklijke Marechaussee, legernummer 19.12.29.008, behorende tot bovengenoemde
Brigade, mij als Commandant van een bevolen Garnizoenspatrouille
le en vergezeld van .... H S H L B D,dpl. Marechaussee 4e
klasse, legernummer 33.04.29.200, behorende tot de 4e Divisie
Marechaussee Compagnie te Harderwijk, op de openbare weg de
Leuvenumseweg te en in de bebouwde kom der gemeente Ermelo. Op
tijd en plaats voormeld zag ik dat een mij onbekend, in de uniform der Koninklijke Landmacht (zomertenue) gekleed persoon
op genoemde weg liep, terwijl hij de mouwen van zijn overhemd
tot boven de ellebogen had opgerold. Bedoelde persoon was vergezeld van een vrouwspersoon, die hij een zijner armen om de
hals had geslagen. Terwijl bedoeld persoon, die de rangonder-
scheidingstekenen van korporaal droeg, alzo in deze weinig
krijgstuchtelijke houding op de openbare weg voortliep, zulks
ten aanschouwe van enige tientallen militairen die zich bij de
IJssalon aldaar ophielden, gaf ik hem opdracht zich bij mij te
melden, door hem te zeggen: "Militair komt U even hier." Het
was mijn bedoeling hem buiten tegenwoordigheid van het meisje
terzijde te nemen, teneinde hem zijn tenue in orde te laten
brengen. Inatede van het meisje achter te laten, kwam hij op
mij toe, terwijl hij dat meisjenog steeds met zijn arm om haar
hals vasthield. Ik vroeg hem waarom hij zijn meisje niet even
terzijde gelaten had, waarop hij mij zijn geringde vinger voor-
hield en mij toevoegde: "Pardon, ik ben verloofd; ik ben niet
gewend dat men mijn verloofde "meisje" noemt."------------------
     Bedoelde persoon verklaarde mij dat hij wel wist dat het
buiten dienst- of oefenverband verboden is de mouwen van het
overhemd opgerold te hebben. Toen ik hem rapport aanzegde, zeide hij: "Ik zie het rapport dan wel, sergeant. Het komt bij
mij binnen, ziet U. Ik ben namelijk administrateur." Toen ik
hem zeide dat ik wel zou zorgen dat hij dat rapport niet in
handen kreeg, vertrouwde hij mij toe dat hij het heus wel zou
doorzenden. Hij gaf mij desgevraagd op te zijn genaamd: - - - -
FRITS EVENBLIJ, legernummer 33.05.03.094, in werkelijke dienst
als dienstplichtig korporaal bij de 152ste Zware Transport Compagnie, gelegerd in de legerplaats Ermelo.---------------------
     Nadat hij in mijn opdracht zijn overhemdsmouwen naar onlaag
had gedaan en ik hem had gezegd dat hij zijn weg kon vervolgen,
liep hij, zonder de groet te brengen van mij weg met de woor-
den:"Goedenavond heren." Ik heb hem hierop teruggeroepen en
nadat ik hem had gezegd dit niet zo gewend te zijn, salueerde
hij overdreven model, waarbij hij vroeg:"Is er nog iets van Uw
orders, sergeant," ofschoon ik hem telkenmale dat hij mij aan-
sprak als sergeant, had gecorrigeerd, dat hij mij met wacht-
meester diende aan te spreken. Het kwam mij, rapporteur voor,
dat bedoelde korporaal deze tegenstrevige houding aannam uit
wraak over zijn staande houding. - - - - - - - - - - - - - - -
     Zijn naamopgave heb ik vergeleken met het in zijn bezit
zijnde militaire identiteitsbewijs en in orde bevonden. - - - -
                              Harderwijk, 22 Juni 1954.
                              De Wachtmeester le klasse,
                                        V.G.
                                        -Gezien-

225

13

THE DECISION

1955 I had them. The documents proving I'd finally been released from my service to the Royal Netherlands Army. I rechecked that they were safely in my briefcase—just in case they changed their mind.

My former employer gave me my old job back, and the Family Verbeek was happy to receive my rental payments again. It was almost as if those 22 months hadn't happened. I was ecstatic about leaving the former days behind and hoped for a wonderful future. First, I pondered, laying a few ghosts to rest might be good. Maybe find out if some things in my past were as bad as I remembered. Perhaps they weren't unforgivable after all.

Jan, wearing his military uniform much more comfortably than I ever did, settled back in the chair in my small room and crossed his legs at the ankles. "You know, I enjoy the army—maybe because I'm not as obstinate as you. No time in solitary for me! Even better, Mama told me that since I'm an adult, she'll have no more control over me. About time!"

I grinned and winked. "And because you're living on base, you don't even have to pay her extortionate rent."

"Never again," my brother vowed before helping himself to another *speculaasje*.

"Hey Jan, do you ever think about our childhood?"

"*Nee*, not if I can help it. Naturally, I don't remember the Congo. And the rest is too awful to contemplate." His eyes became unfocused as his thoughts traveled into the past.

I scratched my head. "Really? Although the sisters at *het kindertehuis* were strict, and the war was, of course, terrible, I sometimes wonder if life in Driebergen wasn't as bad as we thought."

Jan jumped to his feet, his face red and his fists clenched. "Stop! Don't talk about it! There's nothing to say. Ever!"

I raised my eyebrows in surprise but kept going. "Well, Zuster Deenik…"

Jan slammed his hand onto my table, making it jump. "I'll leave, Frits. I will!"

"Okay, okay. Let's talk about women—do you have a girlfriend yet? Maybe a rich one to make Moeder happy?"

Jan punched me in the shoulder, and we were back to normal. Except I now knew that, for Jan, our time at *het kindertehuis* had been indescribably horrible. Perhaps watching someone you love being abused is worse than receiving the blows yourself.

Next, I decided it was high time to address Papa's death. While Meta and I were having dinner with Moeder and Vader, I broached the topic. "Moeder, I'd like to show Meta Papa's grave. Where is it?"

Moeder paused to finish chewing and swallowing her bite of potato. "I don't know."

"What do you mean? You arranged his burial, didn't you?" I felt Meta take my hand under the table as my eyebrows met in the middle of my forehead.

"Yes, as his widow, I had to, you know. But I've never visited the grave and honestly don't know where it is. Remember, we were in the middle of a war." Moeder took a sip of wine before delicately wiping her lips.

Feeling my face flush with anger, I urgently continued my unwelcome questioning. "Well, do you know in which cemetery they buried *your husband*?"

Moeder's nostrils flared. "Of course: Westduin. If you were to ask them, I'm sure they'd be able to tell you where he's buried. Now, this is most unsuitable as a dinnertime conversation. Let's change the subject." She promptly stuck a piece of meat in her mouth, and I knew further questions were useless.

Although it was July, the clouds hid the sun, and the wind whipped Meta's hair around her face while we spoke with the Westduin cemetery official.

"Meneer Evenblij is buried somewhere between these three gravestones." He pointed to a map. "But, with this place being so overcrowded, five others are buried there, too. It'd be impossible to say which body is him."

"*Dank u wel*, meneer."

"You're lucky. We 'shake' the pauper's graves every ten years and put the bodies in a common grave, but we haven't done that section yet."

Holding hands, Meta and I set off toward where he'd indicated, me clutching the paper on which I'd jotted the exact location.

"Look, I think this is where he meant!" Meta stood between several large gravestones. There was nothing that said 'Frederik Evenblij 1899-1942,' but we knew there wouldn't be.

"*Ja*, this looks like the right place." I pocketed the map before bending down to touch the soil, utterly lost in the memories of how Papa loved me. My eyes welled up with tears; I still missed him so much.

Meanwhile, Meta laid the flowers she'd picked in the middle of the grave. Then she carefully walked toward where we figured his head would be, clutching the daffodil bulbs she'd bought and stashed in her pockets. I knew she wanted to plant them there. "I really hate walking on graves. It feels like a sacrilege…aahh!"

I was startled, and my heart leaped into my throat. Meta, her face the color of snow, was now standing with her left leg in Papa's grave. It seemed the splintering wood of the coffin directly beneath the soil couldn't hold her weight.

"Frits, my foot is stuck!" Meta shook her leg frantically.

I quickly pulled my trembling fiancé up out of the grave, and she began sobbing out her terror. "I…my…foot was…in someone's chest! The ribs…fell apart when…you pulled me out!"

Putting my arm around her, I led Meta away from the gravesite. "Papa was a k…k…kind man. Don't worry. He didn't mind." My joke fell flat. Very flat.

A few months later, we returned to find that the city had indeed dug up all the graves in that area of the cemetery. They'd placed the bones in a large hole surrounded by a wooden fence. As we walked away with our heads bowed, I realized that Papa's last resting place was now a little like those of my cousins and Keetie. The official record of his burial was expunged; his memory was now nowhere except in my heart.

Meta, peeking up to see my reddened eyes, whispered, "What was in that grave wasn't him; it was just his body."

I took a deep breath before winking at her. "Minus a rib or two."

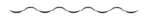

Meta, Sieglinde, Lou, and I crowded into my new home, a little room on the Namensestraat, number 37. This place also had neither a kitchen nor a private bathroom nor would the *zedenpolitie* permit Meta and me to meet there alone. But it was within walking distance of Meta's house, and that was enough.

Sieglinde and Meta's knitting needles provided background rhythm to our conversation. They were making an outfit for their new nephew, Frank, who'd just been born to Corrie and Piet. Lou and I were playing chess.

"I think maybe you should make the shorts bigger, Siegie. He'll grow fast!"

"*Ja*, but he's still pretty tiny. He doesn't even know how to smile!"

Meta's eyes became unfocused, and she put her knitting down. "Do you think Corrie is happy?"

"She should be. She's married to the man she loves."

"*Ja*, but they had to start their marriage living with Pappa and Mamma! And now that Frank is born, they live in that nasty apartment behind the greengrocer. That's not much better. I'd hate it." Meta glanced my way.

I winked and grinned at her, causing her cheeks to turn a pretty pink. "Me, too. No vegetables for me!"

"That's not what I meant, Frits, and you know it!" Meta turned to her sister again. "I so envy you and Lou, Siegie, getting married in only five months. Frits and I haven't even set a date! And we were engaged first…"

Sieglinde, who was bent over her knitting, lifted her head. "Maybe because you're picky about where you'll live. You know the Netherlands doesn't have housing."

I joined in. "It's so aggravating. We all were bombed, but the world decided to rebuild Germany preferentially."

"And they're the ones who caused the problem!" Lou growled.

The pace of Meta's knitting increased as she murmured, "I suspect that's just the excuse being used. After all, we didn't see much progress last time we visited Germany, and that was three years after the war ended."

Lou's eyes narrowed fiercely. "Perhaps the truth is we don't get houses because wealthy immigrants from Indonesia are given priority over people who already live here."

Meta sighed. "It's always that way. The rich get what they want; the poor get nothing." I remembered her indignation about how wealthy children in catechism class were given chocolates while she only received *zuurtjes* and grinned.

"They're living in camps! Some have been there for years." Sieglinde's eyes filled with tears. "How desperate do you need to be to do that? *Nee,* I'd rather live with a parent."

"Sieglinde, I seem to remember that Lou and you were considering emigrating at one point. What changed your mind?" I asked.

Sieglinde bit her lip. "Moving away from family is frightening. Lou and I would rather stay where they speak Dutch! Besides, we're not fussy, are we, Lou?" He nodded, and she continued. "We're okay with living in a tiny room with his mother. It's better than living apart."

Meta scoffed. "We'll see what you say next year! Others seem to have survived emigration. I heard that Meneer Popa and his family moved to Australia. Leo van Kruijsen is going there, too."

"Good for them. We're staying here," Sieglinde retorted.

"Scaredy-cat!" Meta whispered under her breath.

Getting to my feet, I quickly changed the subject. "What do you all say that we go for a walk in the dunes?"

The following Saturday, Meta invited me to have dinner with her family. I cycled the short distance to Leeuwardensestraat, put my hand through the mail slot, and pulled the rope to open the door. "Meti, I'm here."

My gorgeous fiancé ran down the stairs as I ascended them two at a time. We met halfway, and she flung herself into my arms. "Frits, come on up." Meta took my hand and started up the stairs. "Dinner is almost ready. Here, take off your coat—I'll hang it up." She pulled me into the kitchen and continued, now whispering, "Guess what? My cousin Albertine and her fiancé Henk are here. They're also considering moving. Of course, Tante Agnes is hoping her only child won't move. Pappa said he'd like it if we stayed near, too, but he also said he'd like us to have a good life. So…"

I grinned, marveling at how Meta could keep both sides of a conversation going. "I have news, too. I've applied to the NAHV, the firm that employed my father. That work would be in Belgium, so your pappa may get his wish. Unless they send us to the Congo."

Meta bit her lip. "Wow. Africa. It'd be so far from here. Still, at least we'd be together. Come on!" She tugged me into the living room, which was filled with Pappa's cigarette smoke.

"What's that? You're thinking of taking my daughter to the Congo?" Clearly, Pappa had good hearing. "Is it safe? Maybe France would be better."

I frowned. "France?"

"I heard it just after the war ended, but it might still be true. Then, France was so desperate for workers that it offered free land to anyone who agreed to be a farmer. I considered it myself, but we have a house. And I don't know how to farm. You're young. You could learn. What would you think about that, Frits? At least, it wouldn't be on the other side of the world."

I shook my head. "I prefer numbers to chickens, Meneer Bisschop. But maybe we'll get lucky and be given a place here." I knew about the Dutch rule that a couple couldn't get an apartment unless their ages add up to 65 and they have a baby, but a man can hope.

Later, over dishes, Meta's shoulders slumped. "Maybe we should get married and each live in our own places: me with my parents and you in your room. At least we could go on vacation together."

"I don't know. I guess it'd be better than this. There's no doubt that we've been engaged for too long."

Meta sighed, "Much too long."

"Okay, let's set the date. Does December 2 seem good?"

Meta's eyes were red, but she agreed. "Yes. Let's go tell my parents we made our decision."

As Meta surreptitiously kissed me goodbye that evening, she slipped a poem into my hands. After reading it with tears obscuring my vision, I tucked it in a folder along with Papa's letters to be kept forever.

Het was op een Zaterdagavond in Maart,	It was on a Saturday evening in March,
Op dansles leerde een jongen een meisje kennen,	At dance class, a boy met a girl,
Zijn hart ontvlamde; zij was zijn liefde waard,	His heart inflamed; she was worthy of his love,
Hij wilde haar dat echter niet bekennen.	However, he didn't want to admit it to her.
Maar een hart laat zich nu eenmaal niet dwingen,	But a heart cannot be controlled,
Amor won alweer terrein,	Love was gaining ground again,
Zijn hart bleef haar liefheid bezingen,	His heart kept singing her sweetness,
Hij wilde haar charmante ridder zijn.	

He wanted to be her charming knight.

Op 16 Juli moest zij echter examen doen,
Daardoor raakte Don Juan wat van streek,
Hij nam een hele vrije dag toen,
Waarin hij niet van haar zijde week.

On July 16, she had to take an exam,
This somewhat upset the lover,
He took a whole day off,
in which he did not leave her side.

Tussen de middag had ze vrij om te eten,
En ze was opgelucht dat het zo goed was gegaan,
Desondanks kon ze toch van spanning niet eten,
Hij dacht verontrust, "Wat nu gedaan?"

At noon she was free to eat,
She was relieved it had gone so well,
Still, she couldn't eat for excitement,
He thought, troubled, "What should we do now?"

Plotseling kreeg hij een reuze idee,
Hij ging met haar wandelen in het bos,
Zij ging gewillig met hem mee,
Toen kwam ook haar hartje langzaam los.

Suddenly he had a great idea,
He took her for a walk in the woods,
She willingly went with him,
Then her heart slowly began to loosen.

Hij leidde haar naar een overschaduwde bank,
Daar gingen ze zitten, hand-in-hand,
Zijn hart klopte ontstuimig, hard!
Zijn liefde geleek een grote brand.

He led her to a shady bench
There they sat, hand-in-hand,
His heart was beating loudly,
His love burnt like a great fire.

Hij pakte het meisje van zijn dromen,
En omhelsde haar en kuste op haar mond,

He took the girl of his dreams,
Held her close and kissed her mouth,
She did not try to escape his kiss,

Zij probeerde niet aan zijn kus to
ontkomen,
Er heerste een diepe stilte in het
rond.

There was a deep silence all
around,

Haar hart begon van liefde snel
te kloppen,
Zij schonk hem haar hart en haar
ziel,
Iets nieuws en schoons werd toen
geboren,
Een schone dageraad begon te
gloren.

Her heart began to beat fast
with love,
She gave him her heart and her
soul,
Something new and beautiful
was born,
A fair morn began to dawn.

Opeens was de stilte rondom
verbroken,
De vogels jubelden luide hun
lied,
Blij, dat een nieuwe liefde was
ontloken,
De bomen ruisten met hun blaren
een welkomstlied.

Suddenly the silence all
around was broken,
The birds shouted aloud in
their song,
Glad a new love had
blossomed,
The trees rustled welcome
with their leaves.

Nog een vreugde wachte het
jonge stel,
Want aan het eind van deze
middag,
Hoorden zij van haar examen de
uitslag,
Zij was geslaagd als éen van de
besten nog wel!

Another joy awaited the
young couple,
Because at the end of the
afternoon,
They heard the results of her
exam,
She passed as one of the best
yet!

Die avond vierde men toen een
feest,
Gelach en muziek weerklonken
overall,
Maar de jonge geliefden genoten
het meest,
Van hun geluk, het grote bezit van
elkamder.

That night they celebrated
with a party,
Laughter and music echoed
everywhere,
But the young lovers enjoyed
the most,
Their joy at being each other's
great possession.

233

Veertien maanden later verloofden zij zich,
Hij was toen een fiere soldaat.
Zij droeg een jurk, als de hemel zo blauw,
Hij was op zijn meiske so trots als een pauw.

Fourteen months later they got engaged,
He was then a proud soldier.
She wore a dress like the sky so blue,
He was as proud as a peacock of his girl.

Vandaag is het nu twee jaar geleden,
Dat ik beloofde je vrouw te zijn,
Nu heb ik slechts éen enkele bede,
Dat is gelukkig met jou getrouwd te zijn.

Today it is now two years ago,
That I promised to be your wife,
Now I only have a single prayer,
That's to be lucky enough to be married to you.

Ik hoop een zonnetje te zijn in je leven,
Geheel mijn liefde zal ik je geven.
Ik wil je maken tot de gelukkigste man;
Freddy, ik zal alles doen wat ik kan.

I hope to be a ray of sunshine in your life,
All my love I will give to you.
I want to make you the happiest man;
Freddy, I'll do everything I can.

Als symbool van onze liefde,
Liet ik een wijnglas voor je maken,
Dat je daaruit altijd
Zoete vreugde mag smaken.

As a symbol of our love,
I drew you a wine glass,
That you may always taste
Sweet joy from it.

~~~~~~~~~~

1956 On a beautiful day in May, Sieglinde and Lou were married in a modest ceremony attended only by family. After gazing at her sister's radiant face and Lou's shining eyes, Meta turned to me. "Oh, I wish it were our turn! We've been waiting forever and ever!"

"*Ja,* four years is a very long time." I stroked her soft cheek before continuing, "But I'm pretty sure you wouldn't want to live with Moeder and Vader."

We'd recently received news that a home in the Netherlands would be available for us when I turned 75. Worse, the NAHV had turned me down.

Meta's blue eyes filled with tears. "Corrie is so happy with her baby—he's toddling now—but I wonder if it'll ever happen for us. This waiting is killing me! You're right. Your mother's place would be terrible, but maybe living with Mamma and Pappa wouldn't be so bad. They have a spare bedroom now."

I took Meta's hands. "Be patient. Something will turn up. I just know it." I dug a wrinkled piece of paper out of my pocket. "Here. I wrote out the hymn that always meant so much to me. Read it whenever you're plagued with worries."

As Meta took the paper from my hand, I whispered the first lines from memory. "Whatever the future may bring, the Lord's hand is leading me."

Meta began reading and then gave a little jump. "Look here, Frits. It talks about unknown lands. Maybe God *is* telling us something. Let's trust Him and cancel the December wedding. I don't want to start out living separately. Do you?"

"*Nee,* but are you sure? I mean, something will probably come through. But who knows? We may end up on the other side of the world!" My voice betrayed my enthusiasm. I had no ties to the Netherlands and loved an adventure.

Meta's lower lip trembled as the penny dropped. "I'd follow you anywhere, and it does seem like maybe the Lord is leading us, but…Mamma, Pappa, the sea…"

My hands were twirling with excitement. "I get it, schatje. Scheveningen is your home. But what choice do we have? And the hymn…"

"*Ja,* and it'd be hard to start a family with my parents in the room next door…" Meta stared into space before straightening her shoulders and lifting her chin. "I agree. Let's cancel the December wedding."

"So, we pursue emigration?" I quickly stuffed my dancing hands into my pockets.

Meta gently pulled them out. "Freddy, I love you. Your hands don't bother me." She continued, "About emigrating. It pretty much runs in Mamma's family: Poland to Germany to the Netherlands. You know, even Pappa's family was originally from France. I'm every bit as brave as they are, and I've always dreamed of traveling…"

My heart swelled. My fiancé was a slip of a girl with the courage of a lion. I was sure I didn't deserve her, but I hoped she wouldn't figure that out anytime soon.

The next day, I stopped by the government office to pick up more information. The papers explained that the Dutch government would give emigres three times the taxes they paid in the previous year to help them move. Unfortunately, I'd been in the army earning peanuts then, so the money provided wouldn't be much help. But I was earning now, and I could save.

Once at Meta's house, I spread the papers I'd gathered over the dining table. Pappa was at work, and Mamma and Sieglinde were singing in the kitchen. "Here, look, Meta. It says we could go to the USA. I've always wanted to live there!"

"Yes, but the requirements!" She summarized what she was reading. "You need to win the lottery, have a sponsor, or be wealthy enough to start a business with two American employees. The last two sure aren't going to happen for us, and the lottery is unlikely."

I chuckled. "It seems the good old USA doesn't want us."

Meta looked into my eyes. "But you'd really like to move there, wouldn't you? I know it's your dream. Why don't you put our names down for the lottery? Just in case."

"It couldn't hurt and doesn't cost. Now, what about Australia or New Zealand? Kangaroos and wallabies, you know." I waggled my eyebrows.

"Those are too far away. I'd never see my family again!"

Mamma came into the room while drying her hands. "Agnes told me Australia has a job and housing shortage. Albertine and Henk decided against going there because immigrants have to live in a camp for three or four years before finding a home."

Meta took the pen out of my hand and firmly scratched through Australia and New Zealand.

South Africa was next on the list. I tapped my finger against my lower lip. "Personally, I don't like this option. It's beautiful, but there's so much unrest! One of my work colleagues told me he and his wife moved there and had to return. Apartheid, strikes, revolts, and racial tension. We've been through a war already. I've had enough violence to last a lifetime!"

Meta nodded as she crossed out South Africa. "Not the place for us."

We gazed at what was left. "Well, Metì, it seems we'll be emigrating to Canada. It has j…j…jobs, houses, and snow. Lots of snow. What could be better?"

Meta shrugged. "It's not as if we never get snow and ice here! Let's fill in the paperwork and see what happens."

A couple of months later, after medical examinations, which revealed I had tuberculosis-consistent changes to my lungs but was no longer contagious, we received permission to move. Now, we had to tell our families that it was really going to happen.

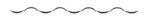

I looked around the crowded dining table. When we told Meta's parents we had an announcement, they invited Corrie, Piet, Sieglinde, and Lou to join us for dinner. Ronald, who was only 11, still lived at home, and Frank was asleep upstairs. After Mamma served up the *hutspot* and gravy, Meta took my hand under the table.

I cleared my throat. "Umm, we received news this week. The government has approved our move to C…C…Canada. Here's the letter."

Silence fell. Eventually, Pappa reached out for Meta and my hands. "Congratulations." His voice stuttered and died.

I looked around the table, shocked to see tears in his and Mamma's, Corrie's, and Sieglinde's eyes.

Meta saw them, too. "Be happy for us. And don't worry. We'll write and even visit."

"I'll start saving now," Pappa whispered.

Telling my family was very different. Vader was impassive, as usual, just eating in silence. Jan wasn't there. Moeder immediately asked about our travel arrangements.

"Most of the people we've asked recommend the ship, the *Grote Beer*. It only takes five days to get there, and it's big enough to be safe."

"Oh, no! That's a bad idea." Moeder frowned. "I recommend you take a smaller boat. Much more luxurious. And, when there are fewer passengers, you get to eat with the captain every night!"

Meta and I exchanged glances. We didn't care how we got to Canada, and we certainly had no aspirations to have dinner with captains. But Moeder was so insistent that we later decided to do as she suggested.

Moeder continued. "When you get there, you'll need a bit of help. I remember moving to a different country as a newlywed! It's not easy, and your father had a job. You won't. I have a third cousin in Toronto, Timon Van Vliet, and his wife, Hanneke. They might help. I'll write him and tell him to expect your letter."

"*Dank u wel*, Moeder." Although we'd not heard a word about her missing me, at least she was helping with the practical arrangements.

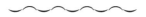

With so many significant life changes on the horizon, I felt restless. "Meti, how about we get away for a few days? Our last chance to relax before the craziness of preparing for emigration begins in earnest."

"And our wedding!"

"Of course. But going away?"

"That sounds wonderful. Where should we go?"

"How about Limburg? The Nationaal Park De Maasduinen is beautiful. We could get a bed and breakfast for a few days—two rooms, of course. Don't want to upset the *zedenpolitie* now that we're so near to being legal."

Meta blushed at my wink. "I've got some money saved, but not much. How about you?"

"Same. But this'll be worth it. We can take our bikes on the train down and then slowly bicycle back here."

"Amazing! Just the two of us for days!"

"And we can use the time to figure out who we'll be inviting to our wedding, where we'll go for our honeymoon, and what we need to pack for Canada."

Meta did a twirl. "You can do that. I'm going to enjoy myself. That's all."

I grinned. My fiancé was a master at procrastination and pretty much the opposite of Moeder, who loved organizing and practicalities more, it seemed, than people.

Suddenly, Meta's face grew solemn. "Hey, Freddy, I have a request. I know you hate the Catholic church, but we're going to be away over a Sunday. How about if I go to a Protestant one? Will you come then? Faith is important to me, and we're going to be married."

I heaved a huge sigh. "Fine, yes. I'll come to a Protestant church."

"Yay!" Meta's eyes shone, and I was glad I'd agreed to her request.

But, when Sunday came, I remembered how her Catholic friends had treated me and how God had allowed Keetie to be murdered.

Over morning coffee and *boterhammen* at the bed and breakfast, Meta listed a couple of nearby churches. "Which one should we go to?"

"I'm not going."

"What? You promised!" Meta's eyes were huge in her pale face.

Sliding my chair back so vigorously that it fell over, I stood. "Don't force me!"

"But…"

My fists clenched as, heedless of the attention we were drawing; I ground out with stiff lips. "No!"

"Frits…*alsjeblieft*!" Tears sprung from Meta's eyes.

"*Nee*. I'm not accountable to you. Stop."

Once again, Meta backed down. We didn't go. But it didn't feel good.

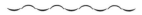

When we came home, the preparations had to begin in earnest. I investigated transport and found we could only afford a freighter: the *Prins Willem II*. There would be seven passengers, including us. Surely, that would please Moeder, especially if we were invited to eat with the captain!

Next, I wrote to Meneer Van Vliet, receiving back a very vague offer of help and a job when we arrived. Not great, but better than nothing.

We set our wedding date to May 14, 1957, because the *Prins Willem II* would leave on June 6. That would give us time for a honeymoon, but we also wouldn't have to spend any time apart.

Since we would need every penny we earned, we decided to have a small ceremony in the courthouse. Only our family and closest friends were invited. I knew Jan would disagree, but on my side, that included the Zusters Dermout and Deenik.

Lou, an excellent tailor, began sewing my navy-blue suit from fine wool. It was to be our wedding gift from him and Sieglinde. Meta began hand-sewing her wedding dress, only doing the long seams with Lou's precious sewing machine. I worked overtime trying to earn and save as much as possible. After all, what the government would provide would not even cover the boat fare.

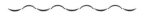

1957 My brow furrowed as I sat at the dining table at Meta's house and calculated how much money we had and how much we still needed. Even with both of us working, when I took out my rent, what I had to give to Moeder, and Meta's contribution to her parents, there was very little left. We'd saved an adequate amount for our honeymoon: I'd budgeted for car rental, hotel, and restaurant. We had sufficient to pay boat fare, and meals were included. I frowned at the page. But was there enough left for when we arrived in Toronto? "Here, Metì, see what I've calculated…"

"Oh, not now! We both took the day off work; the sun is shining, the sky is blue, and I want to get out and have some fun. Come on, let's rent a canoe and paddle down a stream." She pulled on my hand until I stood up and shrugged.

"We might as well. That amount of money won't make much difference."

Meta immediately got busy packing a picnic, all the while chattering about where we'd go and what we'd do. I put a few coins in my pocket, picked up the picnic basket, and we set off for the boat rentals.

"Ooo, this is the life!" Meta leaned back on her hands and lifted her face toward the sun. "That cloud looks just like a fluffy lamb. What do you think?"

I put the paddles down. "It's better that I keep my eye on where we're going than stare at the sky. How about we try our hand at fishing?" The man who'd rented us the canoe had generously thrown in a fishing rod.

"Okay, you put the worm on, and I'll hold the rod."

I chuckled. "Something's wrong with this picture, but fine." I baited the hook while Meta kept her eyes closed. Then, I helped her cast the line. "Now sit quietly so the fish aren't scared away."

She shuddered. "I hope we don't catch a body. Pappa told me the canals are full of them… Eek, what's that?"

I quickly took the line from Meta and reeled it in, pulling out a cucumber. "Not a body. Also, not a fish. Try again."

In no time, Meta caught something else: an old boot. We burst out laughing, and I put the fishing rod away. "Neither the fish nor the bodies are biting today, it seems."

"Not funny! Let's stop here. I'm hungry!" Meta rubbed her stomach. "The meadow looks wonderful for our picnic."

I obediently rowed over to where Meta was indicating. After pulling the canoe onto the bank, I picked up the picnic basket with one hand and helped my fiancé out with the other. The breeze carried the smell of newly cut grass and wildflowers.

"Look, Frits. An apple tree. Let's steal an apple!"

"We'll need two."

"Nope! We need one. You take a bite on that side, and I'll bite from this."

I grinned as a passerby offered to take our picture while we did the deed.

Meta spread out the cloth, and we enjoyed our sandwiches, two more apples, and sparkling lemonade before lying on our backs to finally watch clouds. I felt my eyes drooping, but just then, I heard a snuffling sound followed by Meta's screech. An old goat, after eating the cucumber, was sniffing Meta's hand. Perhaps he hoped for seconds.

This was turning into one scary day. For Meta, anyway.

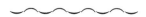

"Freddy, my sisters were so tired after their wedding day that they couldn't enjoy their wedding night. Do you think we could do things differently?"

I winked. "I doubt anything could stop me from enjoying you, but what do you have in mind?"

"I don't want to have the party after our wedding. Let's have one beforehand instead. That way, we can get away early and have a nice dinner together after we're married."

"Great idea. How about having it on the Saturday before our wedding? We could have it at Moeder and Vader's place."

"Yes! Now, what else?" Meta furrowed her brow. "Oh *ja,* I need to buy a dress. I saw one with bronze-colored fabric that shimmers gold. That'd be perfect, especially for dancing. And you can wear your 21st birthday suit. We'll match!"

I grinned. "That sounds beautiful, but you'd look good in anything. Or nothing…"

"Frits!" Meta tucked her hair behind her ear. Then, another thought struck her. "We can invite all our friends and relatives and dance until dawn!" Meta did a twirl to demonstrate before pulling a face. "By then, my toes will be thoroughly flat."

"At least, they'll have time to recover before our wedding…"

Frits and Meta with a goat, 1955. (top)

Papa's unmarked grave, 1955. His remains were moved to a common grave in the same year. (bottom)

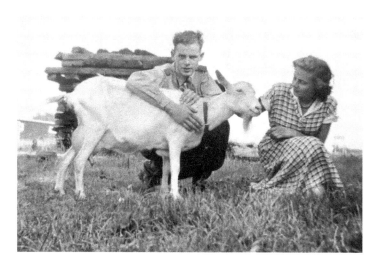

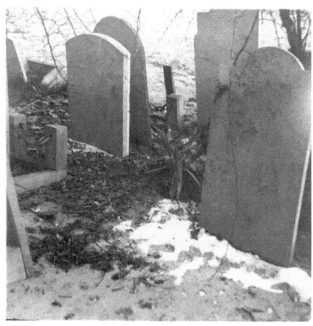

Frits and Meta on a date, 1956. (top)

Meta's love poem to Frits. (bottom)

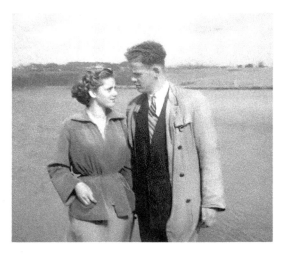

14

THE WEDDING

It was finally here: my wedding day. While getting dressed in my new wedding suit, I thought about the turnaround in my life. Once, I was unwanted and, after Papa's death, pretty much unloved. Now, I knew beyond a shadow of a doubt that Meta adored me. Once, I was abused and neglected. Now, Meta had even ironed and laid out what I should wear today, packing my honeymoon *koffer*, as well. Once, I was angry because Moeder deprived me of my dream of being an electrical engineer. Now, my fondest dream, that of being Meta's husband, would come true. Once, I had to dance to someone else's tune. Now, the most wonderful girl in the world was willingly giving up her rights for the love of me. I was walking on air.

I stood by the window of my little room, waiting for one of the four black chauffeur-driven cars we'd rented to arrive. It would take me the four blocks to Meta's parental home. When I'd grumbled about this ridiculous extravagance, Meta assured me it was necessary. One of the other cars would take Meta's parents, Moeder, and Vader. The third would take Jan and Sieglinde, our witnesses, Piet and Corrie, as well as Ronald. And the last would take the sisters from *het kindertehuis,* Juf van Kempen, and Tante Roo.

There the car was! I snatched up the bridal bouquet, checked if my tie was straight, my shirt tucked in, and my shoes shined, and ran down the stairs.

"Congratulations, Frits! Enjoy!" came the greeting from my landlord as I hurried past.

The uniformed chauffeur jumped out of the car and held the back door open for me, closing it after I went in—a bit like I was royalty. I briefly wished that Papa, Yohan, Mathieu, Keetie, and my cousins' family could see this day, but cleared my mind with a quick shake of my head. Grief wouldn't bring them back; this was Meta's and my day.

The car rolled to a stop outside Meta's home, where I glimpsed the net curtain falling closed. She doubtless saw me coming. I jumped out of the car before the chauffeur could open my door and rang the doorbell with one hand. The bridal bouquet of fragrant stephanotis was in the other. For a few minutes, nothing happened, and my heart pounded in my chest. What if Meta had changed her mind?

The door swung open, and there she was, dressed in all her wedding finery, her eyes shining and her smile lighting up the entire street. I held out my hand with a little bow but couldn't say a word.

"Why thank you, kind sir," Meta twinkled before kissing my cheek.

"C...c...come on. We need to get in the car. The ceremony starts at 11:10."

"Are we late? I was awake until 3:00 am sewing my headdress, so I slept too long this morning." My fiancé often found timekeeping a problem.

"You look gorgeous. And don't worry. They can't start without us, anyway."

In the car, Meta pinned my boutonniere of softly colored freesias onto my lapel. Then, I kept Meta's hand in mine, hardly able to believe that today this person would promise never to leave me. I, in turn, made a silent vow to protect and provide for her for the rest of my days.

Finally, we arrived at the stately City Hall, where the cars with everyone else were waiting. Meta rushed over to Sieglinde. "Did you see the neighbors looking out their windows at us? I'm pretty sure that, after we postponed our wedding, they thought it'd never happen."

Sieglinde, whose swollen abdomen was barely visible under her voluminous dress, giggled, "And still, you know some of them are going to say it happened in too much of a hurry."

I took Meta's hand, knowing full well that she could talk with her sister for hours and never even notice the time go by. "Let's go, schatje."

We entered the gorgeous building, walked up the elegant staircase, and met Cor Houthuis and Harry Kooimans, friends who said they'd take photos. After a few pictures, a waiting usher showed us into a beautifully decorated room with seating for about 50 guests and witnesses. The court officials, a man and a woman, sat behind a table at one end of the room, their position briefly calling to mind the Nazi soldiers in Driebergen. As Meta and I sat in front of our 24 guests, waiting, I forcibly pushed troubling memories from my mind.

At precisely 11:10 am, the lady from the city hall stood and gave a short but delightful talk, none of which I remember today. We went forward to say our vows and exchange the rings, which we'd now had inscribed with our wedding date, and placed them on our left hands. That would signify that we were married. We and our witnesses signed the paperwork. It was done, and it only cost us 12.50 guilders. I resisted the temptation to kiss my wife because it would embarrass her. There would be plenty of kisses later.

Moeder and Vader hosted our wedding lunch, where I had the chance to reconnect with Zusters Dermout and Deenik. Jan adamantly refused to speak to them, but I remembered my vow to forgive. I found them quite pleasant, especially when one is not a small boy.

Eventually, Meta and I set off in our blue rental car. Our first stop would be dinner in Dordrecht.

Meta leaned forward in her seat in the restaurant. "While you were checking on our reservations, I saw the lady next to you looking at you and almost told her, 'You're too late, miss. He just married me this morning!'"

I grinned. "I'm sure you were imagining things. She wasn't interested in me. But I'm glad you're still happy with your decision— even several hours later!"

We honeymooned in Germany, getting back in time to pack the necessities for our new life, including the red radio.

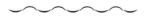

Our families accompanied us on the 6:52 train to Rotterdam, where the Prins Willem II left on its journey to Toronto. I noticed that Jan and most of Meta's family had tears in their eyes. Her mother later told us that her father was sick with grief and cried every day for a year.

Perhaps I should have been sad about saying goodbye to Jan, who I knew would miss me, but I was much too happy and nervous. Meta had been sick to her stomach every morning for a week now, so I knew there was a little, but important, additional reason why we would need a home and jobs quickly. The responsibility almost overwhelmed me.

It was a miserable crossing. The waves were often higher than the deck of the tiny boat, and it was tossed and turned by every one of them. I ate with the captain once or twice, but Meta just fed the sharks, if you understand my meaning.

Making things worse, the boat broke down six times on its way across the Atlantic. Someone had filled it with the wrong engine oil. Every time the boat stood still, the sharks circled enthusiastically. The journey seemed endless.

"Land! I see land!" Meta was standing on the deck, pointing to the horizon.

"Congratulations! The first person to see land gets a commemorative ashtray. Here you are."

"Umm, *bedankt*?" Meta's pale cheeks grew slightly pink as she caught my wink. Why would we, as nonsmokers, need an ashtray?

That night, we were told that the boat wouldn't go to Toronto but to Ottawa. From there, we would be put on a train for Toronto.

Now, it was up to us. By forgiving, I had cut my ties with the past. There was only $30 left in my wallet but I believed the best was yet to come.

Frits and Meta's wedding, May 14, 1957.

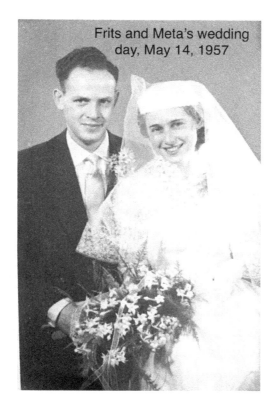

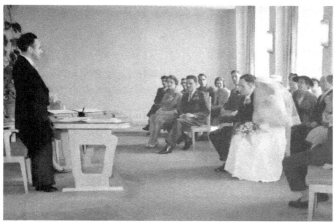

Ticket to the freighter, Prins Willem II. (top)

Saying goodbye on the boat, left to right is Pappa, Moeder, Corrie, Mamma, and Vader. Meta is in the foreground. (bottom)

ORANJE LIJN

(MAATSCHAPPIJ ZEETRANSPORT) N.V.
ROTTERDAM

HOOFDAGENTEN: ANTHONY VEDER & CO. - ROTTERDAM

BEWIJS VAN TOEGANG

voor .... persoon

personen

tot LOODS I IJSELHAVEN

tot M.S. PRINS WILLEM II

Naam van houder: *Mr and Mrs F. Evenblij*

Datum : −6. JUN. 1957

Dit bewijs — dat te allen tijde kan worden ingetrokken — is, mits voorzien van de contrôle-strook, uitsluitend geldig op de datum erop vermeld. Op verzoek is de houder verplicht dit bewijs te tonen.

ROKEN IN DE LOODS EN OP HET TERREIN IS VERBODEN.

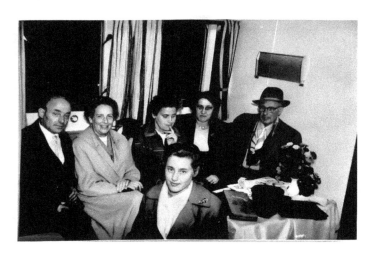

15

THE EPILOGUE

Frits

Frits and Meta arrived in Toronto with few belongings and no spoken English. But, with the help of the van Vliets, both found jobs almost immediately. They learned English by using that language exclusively, even when alone.

Their first child, Irene Caroline, who is also the author of this book, was born in January 1958, closely followed by a son, Robert Frits, in October 1959.

Frits and Meta moved to Brantford, Ontario, in 1961, and twin boys Peter Anthony and Michael Alexander joined the family in March 1965. More about this part of Frits and Meta's life can be found in *Ireentje Learns the Hard Way*.

Nine years after they immigrated to Canada, Frits's dream of living in the USA came true. Massey Ferguson, where he was working at the forefront of the use of computers, transferred him to Des Moines, Iowa. The USA initially rejected his application for a work visa since he was born in the Congo. However, because the young couple put their names down for the lottery while still in the Netherlands, officialdom eventually agreed to allow them to move. Provided, that is, that Dutch-born Meta was the "head" of the family. Their youngest daughter, Jody Melinda, was born in Iowa in 1968.

Frits always enjoyed classical music. His family often found him finger-dancing to the strains of Beethoven, Mozart, and the Viennese waltzes while seated in his chair. Caroline fondly remembers sitting next to him while he played the piano, just like he did with Keetie. As a result, with his help, she also learned to play—from the same book he used.

Throughout his life, Frits continued his love affair with swimming, spending vacations on a lake, water skiing, swimming, and boating. Caroline was grateful for his expertise: he saved her from drowning when she was a teen!

What about Frits's consuming interest in electronics? That continued for his whole life. He initially worked with computers when they took up an entire room. He was the first in his neighborhood in England, where the family moved in 1979, to own a PC. Frits invented and used an Excel-type program many years before Microsoft figured it out, and he wrote the software so that Caroline's George Mason University and Northern Virginia Community College students could access her course and their grades online. This was a decade before the development of Canvas and similar online platforms. He even wrote a program for the Department of Defense while Caroline worked at the Uniformed Services University of the Health Sciences, saving the research team weeks of labor again and again. In fact, during all of his life and even after retirement, Frits helped his children, friends, and colleagues by writing and troubleshooting computer programs. Although he never graduated from college, since he needed three more credits when he moved to the USA, Frits ran circles around many who did.

In 1998, Frits visited the Holocaust Museum in Washington, DC, with Caroline. It was there that he first related to her the painful story of his time in Driebergen, particularly the loss of Keetie. Even though he was just a child at the time, he still could not forgive himself for being unable to save her.

The following year, Frits, Meta, and Caroline visited de Woude. There, they met an elderly resident, Tante Mientje, who had witnessed the lightning strikes and fires and remembered him as a teenager. When informed about who he was, she told Frits to leave. He did not feel guilty about that at all!

Frits never forgot his resolution to forgive and forget, and he lived up to it—as much as possible, anyway. His family never heard him say a bad word about Moeder, Vader, the people of de Woude, the sisters, or anyone else whose actions were, humanly speaking, unforgivable. As for the Nazis, well, he just said nothing.

Whether he ever forgave himself for being who he was is a different question. He was well aware that he was, as Moeder said, "difficult." Others might suggest that he was on the spectrum and also suffered from attachment disorder. Once, while on a trip with Caroline, Frits acknowledged he hadn't been a perfect father. She assured him that she forgave him everything and asked him to forgive her, too. He chuckled despite the tear sneaking down his cheek. "There's nothing for me to forgive. But I wish I could change the past." Caroline silently took his hand. There was little she could say.

In the summer of 2017, Frits received the news that he had terminal cancer. His chief concern was for his beloved Meta, and he repeatedly asked for reassurance that his children would take care of her. Secondarily, he worried that his family might leave him—old insecurities came to the fore with a vengeance as a result of his increasing bodily weakness. He needn't have been concerned; his children and grandchildren flocked to be near as often as possible, while Meta could frequently be seen pressing a kiss to his head.

Although Frits continued to acknowledge the existence of a creator, he didn't think God was interested in him. He said he couldn't believe God would forgive and love him. God didn't give up on Frits; three days before he passed, Frits changed his mind. He said "yes" to the loving Lord who'd been waiting patiently.

On October 18, 2017, Frits died peacefully while he lay in bed, and his darling Meta held his hand. On that morning in Dallas, four of his children were in the home, Peter having visited in the prior week. At his funeral, his granddaughter's husband, Jamie Brown, translated and sang his favorite hymn, Wat de Toekomst Brengen Moge. His daughter's husband, Tim Cooper, wrote a song just for Frits. There is little doubt that, despite much suffering, God was with Frits to the end. His brave legacy lives on.

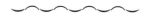

Jan

Jan lived out his days in Den Haag, mainly communicating with Frits via delightful and often hilarious letters and, later, by phone. Jan also visited Frits and his family in England and the USA. Surprisingly for someone profoundly dyslexic, he eventually worked as the Cultural Protection Coordinator at the Ministry of Education, Arts, and Sciences.

Jan married Anne Theresia Dillenius in 1965, and they had two children: Wilfrid and Cilia. Tragically, Anne died in 1976 when the children were still young. Eventually, Jan married again, this time to Hetty, a lovely lady with two children of her own.

Caroline and Meta met with Jan, Hetty, Wilfrid, and Cilia in June 2022. As Meta talked about her memories of Frits, Jan's eyes filled with tears. He loved Frits dearly; the brothers were always close. Jan passed away on October 16, 2022.

Meta, Frits, Hetti and Jan on the beach in Scheveningen, 2010.

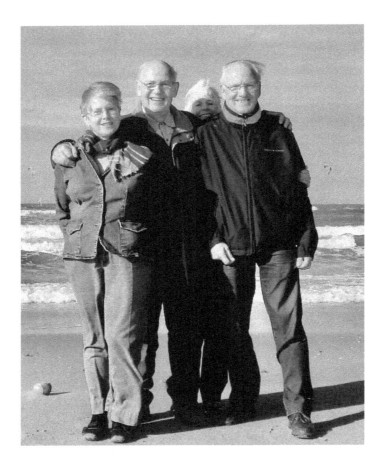

Frits holding Michael and Caroline holding Peter, 1965. (top)

Caroline, Frits, Robert, baby Jody, and Meta in the back. Peter and Michael in the front. Photo taken in Urbandale, Iowa, 1967. (bottom)

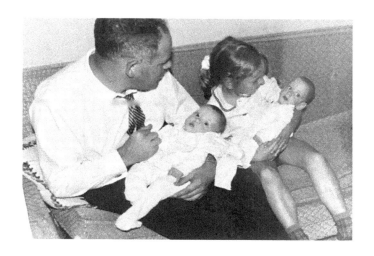

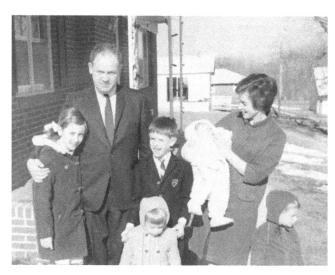

Peter, Michael, Jody, and Robert in the back. Caroline, Meta, and Frits in the front, 2003. (top)

Megan (great-granddaughter), Meta, and Frits, 2010. (bottom)

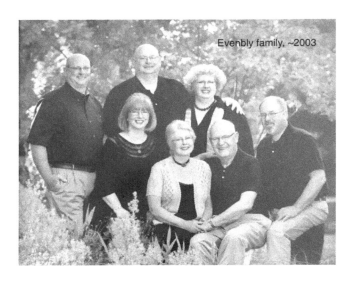

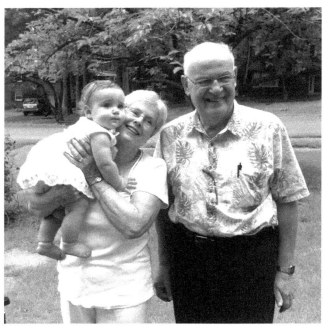

THE POSTSCRIPT

Frits was my only true love. I always aimed to show him how important he was to me. After all, except for Jan, he was special to nobody for most of his childhood. Therefore, I celebrated him, making a big deal of his birthdays, Father's Day, and our anniversary. On his first momentous birthday after our marriage, when we were in our new country, we had tuna fish pie for dinner—a family favorite ever since.

When we were married, a traditional social contract between husbands and wives was still very much in evidence. The husband would work and provide a roof over his family's head, food, and clothing. Frits never shirked this responsibility, no matter how large our family grew. He worked hard both in his jobs and in finding new employment when he was laid off, which happened several times. This was immensely helpful to me, who also suffered much deprivation as a child. After marriage, I always knew we would have enough. I could also be confident that anything that broke would be fixed. I was secure, leaving all the "male" jobs in his hands.

For my part, I tried to make Frits's life easy by doing the tasks he either found difficult or, because of childhood trauma, he refused to do. I cleaned his clothing, packed his suitcases, and, because he was color-blind, even wrote down which tie he should wear with each shirt and suit. Let me assure you that was quite a task during the many times when he had to travel for work!

Of course, most of the time, his job was near where we lived. Then, soon after Frits came home, I had dinner ready. Well, at least I was frying onions, so it seemed like it would be ready soon! The children were cleaned, and the house was tidy. On weekends, we loved to go out, be it on dates or to parties. Another of our chief shared joys was our beautiful home, possibly because of the poverty we experienced during

WWII. I will always remember the pleasure Frits expressed upon seeing my seasonal decorations. I still decorate with him in mind.

Frits truly lived his life by the motto "forgive and forget," but that didn't mean his childhood left him unscathed. I fervently hoped he would heal because of the love I gave him, but in the long run, I couldn't heal his childhood trauma. I couldn't give Frits the love he craved: he wanted his mother's love, as did Jan. Sadly, both men gave up on being loved by her early in adulthood. When their mother died, they were released from the trial of an ongoing relationship but were devastated to know that now she would never recognize their achievements. This was something the brothers dearly desired.

Frits never complained, and the family never knew when he was in pain, even during his final months. It makes me happy to remember that then Frits got his fondest wish: several of his children were with him at all times, and most of his grandchildren visited at least once. One grandson, Jon, brought his baby daughter, Madeleine, over. How Frits loved seeing her commandeer his wheelchair for the use of her toy dog! Whenever one of his children had to leave, I would take Frits to the driveway so he could wave goodbye. His smile would light up his face as they went, but afterward, he would always turn to me and say, "They're coming back, aren't they?"

My husband died peacefully in his sleep, adored not only by his family but by all who knew him. He always said that he wanted to die before I did because he couldn't live without me, and he got his wish. I prayed for Frits daily all his life and, to this day, thank God for his marvelous and merciful rescue of my very tormented husband. We were true partners in life, and I miss him. I love him. I am happy to know that our Father loves him, and I will see him again in heaven.

Meta A. Evenbly
meta@iammeta.org

THE AUTHOR

Dr. I. Caroline Evenbly Crocker is an immigrant born to an immigrant and on for generations. That wanderlust rubbed off. Her parents are Dutch, but she has lived in Canada, Iowa, England, California, Texas, and Virginia. To keep it interesting, she and her British husband adopted a Bulgarian!

Her career has been equally varied. She trained as a scientist specializing in microbiology and immunology. Then, she worked in medical research before teaching cell biology, microbiology, and more at a couple of colleges in VA. After a brief stint as a movie star (seriously!), Caroline founded a nonprofit and learned about websites, newsletters, blogs, and speaking. That wasn't enough of learning new things, so she started a company and took on the dubious pleasures of negotiating with lawyers, writing patents, and finding investors.

And now Caroline is doing what she loves, enjoying her eight grandchildren, gardening, and writing books: adult books, big kid books, little kid books, and even a book on doing microbiology in your kitchen. Nonfiction that reads like fiction.

Nonacademic Books

Brave Face: The Inspiring WWII Memoir of a Dutch/German Child, 2022. The coquel to *Unforgivable,* this historical tale features Frits's wife, Meta, and has a very up-to-date message about war, discrimination, poverty, and even immigration. [https://iammeta.org].

Clemmy Gets a Family, *Clemmy Learns to Talk*, *Clemmy Gets a Job*, and *Clemmy Gets a Sister*, 2023. This series of children's picture books features a brave and endearing bulldog with her very YouTube videos, blog, and website! [https://clemmy.org].

Ireentje Learns the Hard Way, 2017. A humorous children's chapter book about a Dutch immigrant child growing up in Canada [https://ireentje.com].

Growing the Church 101: Being Disciples Who Make Disciples, 2017. A Bible study co-written with the Rt. Rev. Keith Andrews.

Microbiology You Can Do at Home, 2020. A workbook for college and high-school students who love bugs and germs.

Free to Think: No Intelligence Allowed, 2010. Leafcutter Press. A personal memoir written to expand on the movie *Expelled: No Intelligence Allowed*, which starred Ben Stein. The book contains some really cool, if provocative, science.

THE ACKNOWLEDGMENTS

There are so many people who have contributed substantially to this book. If I were to thank all of them adequately, it would be another book!

In first place for my gratitude comes Frits's wife, Meta, known to me as "Mom." She patiently answered my many questions, gave suggestions on the manuscript, unearthed Frits's diary, old photographs, and ancient documents, and explained his father's letters to me. Then, as if that were not enough, she copyedited the entire book.

Thanks also to Jan's daughter, Cilia Evenblij, for sending me her father's written memories and to my Aunt Hetti for allowing the publication of her late husband's story.

I am so grateful to beta readers Mary Springman and Meta Evenbly, who gave fantastic feedback on improving the book, and to Chip Webb, who edited the manuscript. Thanks also to my loving family, husband, children, grandchildren, and more for listening to me talk about my father and providing pointers when needed.

Thanks to Hans Hermans, who provided photos from his Facebook group, enhanced my family photos, and pointed me toward additional information about events in Driebergen. I am also grateful to the members of many Facebook groups (My Dutch heritage, I love my Dutch heritage, Driebergen-Rijsenberg toen & nu, Dutch culture and traditions, All things Dutch) who gave continual feedback and advice. Your input improved the book.

Last but not least, thanks to my son-in-law Jamie Brown, who wrote English lyrics based on Meta's translation of Frits's favorite hymn and sang it at his memorial, and to my brother-in-law, Tim Cooper, who wrote and sang a song dedicated to Frits. Both pieces can be heard on YouTube. https://tinyurl.com/UnforgivableYouTube

More about Frits can be found at https://unforgivable.website.

THE GLOSSARY

Words are Dutch unless otherwise indicated.

Alstublieft, alsjeblieft; s'il vous plaît	please (formal and informal) Dutch; French
Bedankt	thanks
Belgische Congo	Belgian Congo, now Zaire
Boterham(men)	sandwich(es)
Broer(tje)	brother, small brother
Burgemeester	mayor
Dank u wel	thank you (formal)
Der Widerstand, Het Verzet	the Resistance (German, Dutch)
Doe (maar) gewoon	(just) act normal
De dokter/ le docteur	the doctor (Dutch/French)
Doux bébé	sweet baby (French)
(Een) speculaasje	(a) spiced cookie

Garçon	boy (French); condescending form of address
Gemenerik	meanie
Goedenavond, Goedemiddag, Goedemorgen	Good Evening, Good Afternoon, Good Morning
Het bos	the forest
Het is vrede	it is peace
Het kindertehuis	the children's home
Hutspot	Dutch dish made of mashed potatoes, carrots and onions
Ik weet het niet	I don't know
Lieveling	darling
Ja/oui, ja zeker, jawel	yes (Dutch/French); yes, of course or yes, really
Je suis désolé	I'm sorry (French)
Joden/Joods/Joodse	Jews/Jewish
Jongeman	young man
Juffrouw/ Juf	Miss
Kachel	coal-burning stove
De kerk	the church
(De) kindertjes/kinderen	(the) small children/children
Kleine	little

Koffer	suitcase
Lang zal hij leven	Dutch happy birthday song
Lul, stommert, teef	swear words
Ma chérie, mon chérie	my dear (French)
Mama, Mamma, Moeder	mother (upper-class, working-class, formal)
Mattenklopper	carpet beater
Meester	male teacher
Meneer/Monsieur/Herr	Mr. (Dutch/French/German)
Mevrouw/M'dame	Mrs. (Dutch/French)
Mijn	my
Mon petit enfant	my little child (French)
Nee/non/nein	no (Dutch/French/German)
NSBer	Dutch Nazi, traitor
Oma	grandma
Onderduiker	Person in hiding
Oom	uncle
Opa/Grand-père/Großvater	grandfather (Dutch/French/German)
Papa, Pappa, Vader	father (upper-class, working-class, formal)
Poempie	unknown meaning

Schatje	sweetheart
Schweigen (Sie, Allen)	silence (you, everyone)
Tante	aunt
(Ton) petit frère; kleine broertje	(your) little brother (French; Dutch)
Hartelijk gefeliciteerd met je verjaardag	happy birthday
(Vieze rot) Mof/ Moffen	dirty rotten German (slur-word)
Zedenpolitie	morality police
Zugführer	commander (German)
Zuster	sister or nurse
Zuurtjes	sour boiled candies

THE APPENDIX

Beninnk, Aleida Christina (Tante Aleida)	Frits's mother's mother
Bisschop, Corrie	Meta's eldest sister
Bisschop, Meta Antonia (Metí)	Frits's girlfriend, fiancé, wife
Bisschop, Ronald	Meta's younger brother
Bisschop, Sieglinde (Siegie)	Meta's older sister
Bloemist, Rosalie	Jewish friend in Driebergen
De Boer, Unknown	Farmer in de Woude
Deenik, Wilhelmina (Mien)	Nurse at het kindertehuis
Dermout, Suzanna Elisabeth (Suus) (Gemenerik)	Nurse at het kindertehuis
Evenblij, Frederik (Freddie)	Frits's father
Evenblij, Frits (Fritsje, Toni, Freddy)	Frits
Evenblij, Jan (Jean-Jean)	Frits's younger brother

Evenblij, Maria Johanna (Rita) Wallig (Mama, Moeder)	Frits's mother
Flatow, Anni Amalie	Nurse's friend in Driebergen
Flatow, S. Siegbert Werner	Possible betrayer, Driebergen
Goudsmit, Eduard	Frits's mother's fiance
Hermans, Dokter	Doctor in Driebergen
Holst, Lammerdina (Tante Bep)	Nurse in other children's home
Holst, To (Tante To)	Nurse in other children's home
Imaginary, Dirk (Trouble)	Frits's friend in Driebergen
Marijke	Servant in Den Haag
Mathieu	Houseboy in the Congo
Odewald, Herman	Frits's Jewish friend Driebergen
Ouwerkerk, Jacobus (Cobus, Vader)	Frits's stepfather
Scheventanden, Pieter	Jan's foster family's son
Schevetanden, Mevrouw	Jan's foster mother
Sinterklaas	Santa Claus (kind of)
Smit, Dokter	Frits's father's doctor
Tomey, Lou	Meta's sister's fiancé/husband
Tonnon, W.M.	Driebergen mayor during the war
Unknown, Arie	Frits's friend in college
Unknown, Henk	Frits's high school friend

Unknown, Jantje	Autistic child in Driebergen
Fretgezicht, Meester	Head of Concordia College
Van Kempen, Meta	Frits's teacher in Driebergen
Van Zanten, Keet (Keetie)	Close friend in Driebergen (Jewish)
Verbeek, Meneer en Mevrouw	Frits's host family in Scheveningen
Verwaand, Unknown	Administrator Concordia College
Wallig, Baby	Frits's cousin, killed at birth
Wallig, Edith	Frits's cousin
Wallig, Esther Mok (Dicky)	Frits's aunt
Wallig, Hans (Hansje)	Frits's cousin
Wallig, Henri (Hans)	Frits's mother's brother
Wallig, Henri Hartog (Opa)	Frits's mother's father
Wallig, Meriam	Frits's cousin
Wildemast, Hans	Frits's army buddy
Yohan	Houseboy in the Congo

THE SOURCES

Beens, Esther. Zoektocht in Archieven. Oorlog, Verraad en Overlevingsdrang.

Benninck, Marianne (penname for Marie J. Evenblij). 1966. *De Werkelijkheid was Anders*. Kruseman, Den Haag.

Evenblij, Frederik. Letters to his sons.

Evenblij, Frits. Childhood diary, 1946-7.

Evenblij, Frits. Letters to Meta.

Evenblij, Frits. Written 50th-anniversary memories.

Evenblij, Jan. Jeugherinneringen-tot Militaire dienst.

Evenblij, Marie Johanna. Letters to her sons.

Evenbly, Meta. Spoken memories, poems, and written letters.

Family archive. Lists, tickets, calendars, photographs, and more.

Hermans, Hans, Various articles on
https://www.facebook.com/groups/driebergenrijsenburgtoenennu

Jacobsen, R. Joods Monument in Driebergen, Kinderopvanghuis: Deenik en Dermout. http://www.jmind.nl/?page_id=28

Joods Monument. Articles on each of the children who were taken from Driebergen and died. https://www.joodsmonument.nl

National Monument Kamp Vught. https://www.nmkampvught.nl/ontdekken/het-verhaal/vermoord-in-vught/holst-lammerdina-elisabeth/

Dear Reader,

Thank you for reading my book. If you loved it, please help me by posting a review on Amazon, Barnes and Noble, Goodreads, etc. Also, feel free to drop me a line at caroline@ramblingruminations.com. I love to hear from my readers!

Caroline

Printed in the USA
CPSIA information can be obtained
at www.ICGtesting.com
CBHW030847130324
5199CB00006B/4

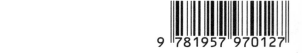